197

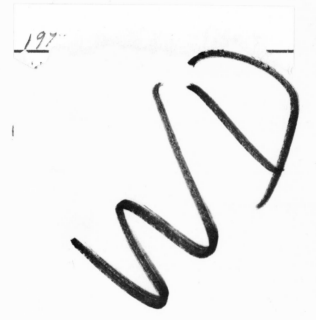

YOU CAN DO IT
FROM
A WHEELCHAIR

YOU CAN DO IT FROM A WHEELCHAIR

ARLENE E. GILBERT

ARLINGTON HOUSE·PUBLISHERS
NEW ROCHELLE, N. Y.

All photos by Don Bennis

Library of Congress Catalog Card Number 73–11578

MANUFACTURED IN THE UNITED STATES OF AMERICA

Library of Congress Cataloging in Publication Data

Gilbert, Arlene E
  You can do it from a wheelchair.

  1. Physically handicapped—Rehabilitation.
I. Title.
RD795.G5   640'.2'408166   73–11578
ISBN 0–87000–218–X

CONTENTS

Introduction   7
1 Basic Wheelchair Information   13
2 Going Out in the World   29
3 Household Arrangements   45
4 Aids   59
5 Meal Preparation   69
6 General Housekeeping   83
7 Floor Care   95
8 Laundry   103
9 Child Care   113
10 Personal Grooming   123
11 Miscellaneous   131
   Appendix: Useful Addresses for the Handicapped 143

105,909

INTRODUCTION

If you're in a wheelchair, you can lead a satisfying, useful life. You can go to movies, swim, bowl and shop. You can also cook, wash clothes, mop floors, and sew.

Maybe you're already thinking, "What does she know about it?" so I'll tell you. I know because I live this kind of life every day. I've been in a wheelchair since 1965 and have four children to look after. Although I stay at home more than most women, I do go out in public and get involved in many activities.

When I originally wrote this book, I was able to do most of my housekeeping with just a little assistance from my family. Now, as I revise certain sections, I can do very little by myself. I have multiple sclerosis and because of this disease and other ailments, my physical condition has gone down. Therefore, you have the advantage of my experiences when I was feeling pretty well and times when I felt considerably less than great.

In this book are sections and sometimes whole chapters which cover basic wheelchair information, various means of transferring to and from a wheelchair, and getting out in the world—driving, shopping, going to church, school or work, voting, groups to join, eating out, attending public gatherings, participating in sports, sightseeing, household arrangements for the wheelchair home, aids to use around the house, taking care of laundry and floors, general housekeeping, meal preparation, child care, personal grooming and miscellaneous other information.

Some of the rehabilitation equipment referred to in this book can be bought at local wheelchair dealers, limb and brace shops, and surgical supply houses or found at rental services. All of these places do not stock the same material so you'll have to inquire in your area what is available.

A good source of different types of bathroom handrails, tub and toilet seats, reachers, and devices for those who can work with only one hand is a Cleo Living Aids catalog. (See the Appendix for address.)

It might be wise to get to know your local hardware store man. Often items not available elsewhere can be found at his place. If you don't see what you're looking for in the store, ask about it. Some things for which there's not a great demand can be ordered by him through his catalogues. If you've got a man as handy and inventive as the one in our neighborhood, he could probably tell you how something you can't find ready-made could be created.

There's no better way to keep up with helps for the handicapped currently on the market than to have a subscription to the magazine for the handicapped, *Accent on Living*. There will be more about this magazine later but right now I'm referring to the information and ads about the latest products and services. Everything from special wheelchair cushions, hand controls for driving and hydraulic lifts to a remote control device for closing draperies, turning on and off lights, TV, appliances, etc. are told about or advertised. Many of the ads invite you to send for brochures or general information. One of these just might provide you with the right answer to a nagging problem.

I sincerely hope that everyone in a wheelchair who reads these pages will find at least a few hints that will make his life easier and happier. *Please note*—Anytime I refer to a company, organization, or service, the address will be listed in the Appendix.

YOU CAN DO IT FROM A WHEELCHAIR

1

BASIC WHEELCHAIR INFORMATION

Since this book is written for wheelchair users, the most logical subject to begin with is wheelchairs.

Everyone's needs differ, of course, but there are so many variations in wheelchairs, there is bound to be one for you. Your doctor and therapists are the people to help you decide what type to get. You can also find out what is available by visiting a wheelchair dealer. If you are undecided which kind of wheelchair would be the most useful for you, rent one (look for wheelchair rental shops in the yellow pages of your telephone book) for a month before getting a permanent chair. If you have used a regular chair in the hospital, for example, rent one with detachable desk arms and removable legrests.

First of all, there is the universal chair with standard, stationary arms and legrests. This one is fine for people who do not need to be in a chair constantly, such as those who are able to walk around the house but must ride when going any distance. It is also all right for those who know they are not going to need one for very long. Almost everyone else, though, has problems which require special features on a wheelchair.

One kind of special chair is designed for one-handed control, such as is needed for some stroke patients. On these, both handrims are on the same side, either right or left.

Chairs especially for leg amputees are available. This type has the wheels arranged a little differently than on most chairs to compensate for the weight loss.

Small people may want to take advantage of a chair that fits more easily into some areas than the average chair—the narrow adult style. This is not a junior-size built small all over and meant for children, but is narrower than a regular adult chair.

For those with little wheeling strength, there is the motorized chair which runs on batteries. These, however, do cost quite a bit more than manually operated chairs.

When transferring is difficult or impossible to do alone, the zipper back is available. With it, the entire back can be opened.

Removable legrests have so many good points that I consider them essential. Numerous occasions arise when having no legrests on the chair is a distinct advantage. One of them is when the only way you can approach a bathtub is in a forward position. At such a time, you really need swing-away, detachable legrests which can be swung away temporarily or taken off completely. That way you can get right next to the tub. More than once this type of legrest has been helpful to me when sitting at a low table. They can be removed and my feet placed on the floor, thus allowing me to get closer to the table. In addition, if it is a small table occupied by several others, my footrests do not protrude and jab everyone's legs. The most useful time to remove my right legrest is every time I transfer to the toilet. With the legrest off, I avoid the excessive bruising I'm bound to get if it is left on. This is because I move over sideways and am unable to stand on my own at all.

Besides detachable legrests, there are the kind which elevate. An elevated legrest can be raised into different positions, which is a necessity for those who must keep one or both legs raised, such as someone with a leg cast or a person who has a lot of trouble with swelling.

Another part of a wheelchair I highly recommend and could not get along without is the removable desk arm. It should easily be seen how simplified transferring can be when you are able to get directly beside the object you want to transfer to and remove the arm completely. As for the difference in arms—with standard arms you cannot get underneath many tables and desks, especially low ones; you can with desk arms. With removable desk arms, I haven't found any tables or desks I couldn't get under. If you come across a situation like that, though, and have detachable chair arms, you can always take the arms off entirely. See Figure 1 for the difference between the two arms.

A number of accessories for a wheelchair are available from the chair dealer. Just a few of these are a hook-on headrest, safety belt (like an automobile seat belt), and foam rubber cushions, which—once you get used to them

15

—you won't want to be without. Some of these cushions have fabric or vinyl coverings. Mine does not, so I cover it with pillow cases.

To help prevent feet from sliding off the footrests, you can get a loop that fits around the back of the heel or straps across the toes. Some chairs with nonremovable legrests have a strip of webbing such as is found on lawn chairs across both legs for this purpose. I find this type very uncomfortable. My chair has a padded section that fits under each calf. Muscle spasms are a problem for me and even the latter device doesn't keep my feet from jumping off the footrests and trailing on the floor. Still, it is far better than the type of chair which has nothing at all behind the leg.

Years ago wheelchairs were drab and ugly but not anymore. In a hospital, they are often all one unappealing color. However, they do come in all sorts of attractive shades. Mine is a medium blue.

Wheelchairs are not exactly feathers to lift. Mine weighs sixty pounds. My husband does all right with it but when a woman is going to take me somewhere, she usually brings along a companion to help. If the man or woman who will most often have to handle the chair alone finds it too much to manage, you can buy a lightweight model which is only half as heavy.

Special features not already discussed can be put into a chair but it is preferable for a doctor or therapist to prescribe them.

Fabric or vinyl parts of a wheelchair, such as the back, seat or armrests are replaceable through the dealer.

Wheelchairs require little maintenance. Some persons

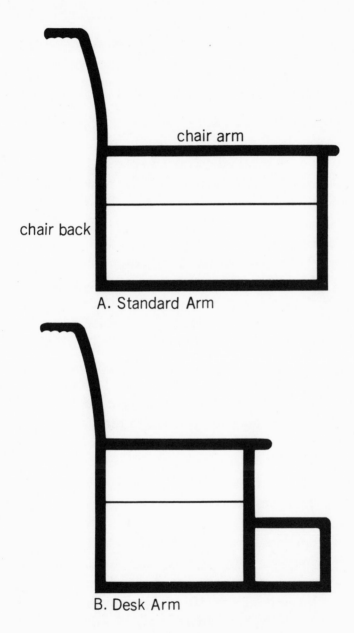

A. Standard Arm

B. Desk Arm

Figure 1. Standard and Desk Wheelchair Arms

can clean their own with a damp rag, some rely on others to do this job. As for lubrication, you will receive a booklet when you buy a new chair telling you where and how often to do this.

Narrow doorways, such as bathrooms usually have, can be a great hindrance to your independence. They can be mastered by a device called a Narrow-matic. It fits on the inner part of your wheelchair and can be removed in seconds. Used regularly, it is worth its cost. Write for literature about this item to Rehabilitation Equipment, Inc.

It may be only occasionally that you need to get through such doorways. Some persons with strong arms can pull up the seat while they are in the chair to make it through the doorway. Another person can do the same thing while standing behind the chair. This is even simpler if the chair has detachable arms because then there are seat straps to pull on.

There should be no doubt about when to lock the chair's brakes—whenever it is safer for the chair to remain in place. That means whenever you are entering or leaving the chair, when you must stay put on an incline, and so forth.

In order to use a wheelchair in the first place, you have to be able to get in and out of it. Learning to transfer the way that suits you best is very important. Ideally, this is learned through practice supervised by a physical therapist. What works for one person may not for another, though, so there is no set way to do it. Those who feel pretty much the same from day to day can find a system and stay with it. With this weird disease of multiple sclerosis, my physical condition and abilities vary from day to day, even from one time of day to another, so I don't transfer exactly the same way every time.

If you have a standard chair with nondetachable arms, this complicates the transferring process. There are three ways I know to get out of bed using this kind of chair. First, you can put the chair at an angle beside the bed, making certain the brakes are locked. Then, sitting on the side of the bed, reach for the farthest armrest with one hand and push off the bed with the other, pulling yourself into the chair. You need strong arms to do this. Don't try it at the start without help.

A second method of getting into this type of chair is to have the chair facing the bed and use a sliding board, sometimes called a bridgeboard, between the bed and chair. The board should be placed far enough onto the seat so it won't fall off (no wider than the chair, obviously) and whatever length is convenient. The board should be sanded smooth before using it. To use, you slide along the board until you reach the seat and, when you are comfortably on it, remove the board.

The third possibility for using a standard wheelchair is by putting a regular chair between it and the bed. In transferring, you slide over to the regular chair, then on to the wheelchair. Naturally, for using either this or the sliding board, you must have plenty of room next to the bed.

To get into a bed from a wheelchair, you reverse the process of getting out, of course.

As far as I am concerned, the only way to get into a chair from a bed is by using a wheelchair with detachable arms parked sideways to the bed. You take the arm next to you off and put it on the bed or, as I do, over one of the handles

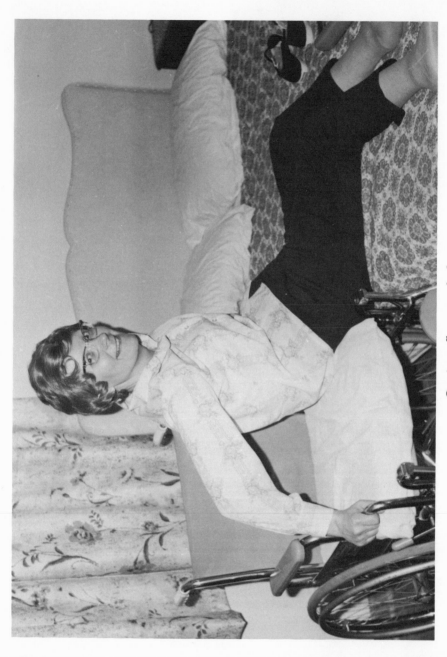

Getting off or on a bed.

that people hold when pushing the chair. The booklet that came with my wheelchair shows a series of pictures of a woman making this transfer, sitting on the side of the bed. She reaches across to the farthest arm and then, pushing off the bed with the other hand, swings herself into the chair. I cannot do it that way myself. I leave my legs out in front of me on the bed, swing over into my chair sideways, and then put my legs down on the footrests. Getting into bed, I get my legs up on the bed first. Here, again, someone who finds such transferring too difficult can use a sliding board.

Another way to transfer to a chair next to a bed with an arm off is to approach it backwards. Reaching behind you with one hand for the wheel and grasping the top of the legrest with the other, you boost yourself onto the seat.

Transferring to the toilet involves much the same routine as getting into bed. A standard wheelchair at an angle, a sliding board, or an extra chair can be used. Again, the room must be large enough for using this equipment. Since standard toilets are three inches lower than most wheelchairs, this can be quite a problem when transferring. If you use a wheelchair cushion, this will add approximately three inches to your height in the chair. That makes you six inches higher than a regular toilet. For the very strong, this is no worry. The rest of us can make up some of the difference in height by getting an elevated seat which attaches to the top of a regular seat. These are reasonably priced and some adjust in height.

Persons not able to get into their bathroom alone may need a commode chair in place of a toilet. Commode chairs and elevated toilet seats can be bought from various places where rehabilitation equipment is sold. Find out what is available at your local surgical supply houses or write to Rehabilitation Equipment, Inc., for brochures or to Cleo Living Aids for a catalog. Some of these items are also available from a Sears catalog, where they are listed under "sickroom supplies."

One thing you really need at the toilet is a handrail. Inquire about the various different types at local surgical supply houses, wheelchair dealers and many rehabilitation equipment companies.

I practically dismantle my chair when transferring to the toilet. Since I approach from the left, I remove the right legrest, which is always in the way, and then take off the right arm. Then, after moving as close as possible to the toilet and locking my chair, I reach across with my right hand to the handrail and behind me with my left hand on the right wheel and throw myself over.

Getting in and out of a tub alone is not wise to attempt until and unless you have practiced the technique with some assistance. The most important thing is to get the wheelchair as close to the tub as possible. If you have detachable arms on your chair and there is room to get beside your tub, you can get into it sideways. If approaching in a forward position when using a chair with stationary legs, you always have to bridge the gap between the chair seat and the tub. When you have removable legs, you can take them off, get almost up to the tub, lift your legs over the top, pull the chair right next to the tub and lock the chair. Then you can move to the edge of the tub, reach to the other side and let yourself down. A grab bar attached to the wall will probably be needed to push on when getting in and out. A number of styles can be bought through local supply houses or from catalogues such as Cleo Living Aids.

If you cannot manage the distance back from the floor of the tub to the edge when getting out, you can take your bath on a small stool set in the water. To prevent slipping, the stool should have suction-crutch tips on the legs, which are available where crutches are sold, and the stool should be set on a bath mat which also has suction cups.

To maintain sitting balance in the tub (if this is a problem) try using a stadium seat or boat seat, minus the hardware. Another way to conquer this difficulty is to bathe with legs crossed in Indian fashion, if that is physically possible. I do this myself, and although I have to hang onto the grab bar until my legs get situated, once they are, even muscle spasms won't throw me over backwards.

When it is impossible for you to take a bath alone and a helper is available but cannot manage you, you might be interested in a patient lift. They can be found in various places which deal with equipment for the handicapped. One source of all types of lifts is Ted Hoyer and Company.

For those who have the combination of a stall shower and the ability to transfer from a wheelchair to a lawn chair set in the shower, this is a way to do it. Also, some of the places dealing with rehabilitation equipment carry shower chairs or commode chairs meant to be used in a shower as well.

There may be times when you will want to transfer to the floor. A mother might like to get next to the bathtub to bathe her small child. Some people want to get down on an exercise mat. Perhaps you have another reason. If getting back into the chair is simple for you, you don't need any hints about doing this. For others, getting from the floor to the chair is a real job. If you are in this category, have you thought of going up gradually such as by sitting on a footstool or other low object before getting into the wheelchair? If this works and you anticipate getting down on the floor often, it is a good idea to have some item designated for this purpose and kept handy for such occasions.

Here is an idea for getting off the floor if, like me, you never are down unless you've fallen out of your wheelchair. I have tried other methods, but this is the *only* way I can get up. The first step of getting back where you belong is to get both you and your chair into the living room. Some people can only get about by crawling or pulling along on the elbows as they do in basic training in the service. I scoot across the floor on my rear, heaving myself forward by pushing down with both hands, leaning forward all the while to keep balanced. As far as moving the chair is concerned, even a small child can push it when empty. If you are alone, you can move it along in front of you a bit, then move yourself, then push the chair again. When empty, a chair rolls easily. Then you park the chair at one side of the sofa, lock it, and back yourself to the opposite side of the sofa. By pushing up the cushion, you have the low sofa on which to pull yourself up; you then proceed to the side where the cushion is and from there to the wheelchair. Your energy may be gone by then, so if you use a wheelchair cushion, you had better remove it before the last step. I have had to do this just a few times and afterwards was so exhausted I had to lie down for a while. I still think it beats lying on the floor until someone arrives home to help, or struggling to make a phone call to ask someone for assistance.

Now that we've gotten back and forth and up and down inside the house, it is time to get in the car and go somewhere. If you have a chair with nondetachable arms, you can park it facing the front seat of the car. If you are on a curb, make certain all wheels are on the curb. You want to *get* into the car, not *fall* into it. For those who do not have the strength to push up and lift themselves across from the chair to the seat of the car, a sliding board can again be put to use.

Using a chair with detachable arms makes transferring so much easier. You get alongside the car and do not have a large gap in between. Some car doors do open farther than others, though, and allow you to get closer. For me, it is best to get my legs in first, then lift the rest of me over onto the seat. Of course, for getting out of the car, you reverse whatever method you used to get in.

If you are able to do your own driving (more about that in the next chapter), one thing you have to remember when getting your wheelchair out of the car is to lock the chair. I know a man who neglected to do this and his chair rolled down an incline. He had to wait in the car helplessly until someone came along to retrieve his chair for him. Luckily, he was on a fairly busy street and did not have to wait long.

Help is needed for getting up and down curbs and stairs. To go up a curb—with you in the street facing the curb— the assistant behind the chair steps on the tilting lever in the back and puts downward pressure on the chair handles

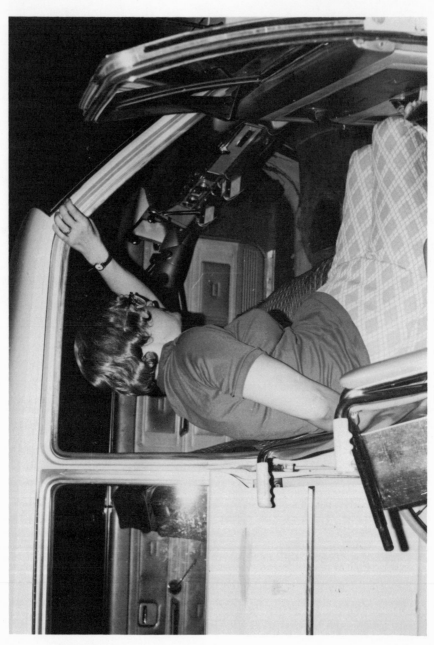

Getting in or out of a car.

until the chair is tilted back on the big wheels. When the small wheels are on the curb, the back is then lifted onto it.

One way to get down from a curb is the opposite of the above with the person in a wheelchair facing the street. The assistant then tilts the chair backwards, pushing down on the tilting levers. This way, he lets the rear wheels down on the street first, then straightens the chair upright. This is fine if people know what they are doing. However, inexperienced people will try to let you down without tilting the chair backwards, and can dump you into the street. I feel it is safer for people to take you down from a curb with your back to the street. Then, of course, they let the back wheels down first.

People always want to help when a wheelchair has to be maneuvered over several steps. Those who have detachable chair arms should be sure no one grabs the arms. They will come off in their hand which will shake them up and not make them the least bit helpful. Tell them to hold the leg or wheel of your chair.

There are a number of wheelchair manufacturers. Three are Everest and Jennings, International Industries, and Rolls Equipment Company.

2

GOING OUT IN THE WORLD

Unless you are completely unable to stay in a wheelchair for any length of time, there are many places you can go in a chair.

Before going to an unfamiliar building, however, it is wise to call and check if it is convenient for a person in a chair. Although old buildings are often ill-suited for a wheelchair, sometimes having many steps and no ramps, many modern buildings do take the handicapped into consideration. These buildings have such things as street level entrances, ramps and elevators. Still, that's only some buildings, not all.

Many cities have guidebooks for the handicapped available for the asking. The one in my city was prepared by the Junior League in cooperation with the local chapter of the Easter Seals Society for Crippled Children and Adults. These booklets list various public places such as stores, restaurants, hotels, office buildings, libraries, cultural, educational, recreational and religious facilities. They describe parking facilities, the width of doorways of both the entrances to the buildings and the restrooms, if there is a phone within reach to those in wheelchairs and whether or not there is an elevator.

In order to get anywhere, of course, you need transportation. Many people must rely on others for this necessity. However, there are plenty of people in wheelchairs who do drive.

It is fairly common knowledge that any good mechanic can rig a car with hand controls. You can have a mechanic obtain these controls and install them or buy them yourself and give them to him to put on. If you buy a new car, there is no problem transferring the controls from the old one. Some brace and limb shops sell hand controls. There are a number of companies that deal in them, and some invite you to write for a brochure about their product. Two such companies are Gresham Driving Aids and the Wells-Engberg Company.

So, actual driving is not the big problem. Getting a wheelchair and getting yourself in and out of the car might very well be more difficult. Since this is a highly individualized undertaking, it is of the most benefit, to someone who wants to find out more about this, to get in touch with a wheelchair driver. I say this because I have talked with about a half dozen persons who drive and each handles it differently. Possibly your doctor or therapist or even friends or acquaintances can refer you to one or more persons who do this. You can also, however, call a large rehabilitation center. Some of them have driver training programs. The lessons are often paid for by the state Division of Vocational Rehabilitation if taking them allows the person in a wheelchair to be more independent. Check with your local office of this state department.

To drive alone, you need a two-door car and must keep your chair behind the front seat while driving. Undoubtedly, there are people who get in on the driver's side, but you avoid clashing with the steering wheel if you enter on the passenger side and slide over to driving position when you have your chair inside.

After getting inside the car, a person with the necessary strength can fold his chair and get it inside with one hand while holding onto the car for balance with the other. Even the not-so-strong figure out ways to accomplish this. Some find that a hydraulic lift attached to the roof of the car is what they need. Information about lifts can be had at some dealers of rehabilitation equipment and wheelchairs. As previously mentioned, all types of lifts are handled by Ted Hoyer and Company.

Several different lifts made for use with a van have been written about or advertised in *Accent on Living* magazine. One even enables the handicapped driver to enter the van himself, then wheel up to the driver's position and drive right from the chair.

A disadvantage of driving alone is when you have car troubles. One man's solution to this is worth considering —a two-way radio so that he's always in touch with some central place. Another help in times of distress are signs which can be hung out of a car window. Some can be obtained through auto clubs or gas stations. Signs that indicate specifically that the driver is handicapped are advertised in some of the literature available from companies which sell hand controls.

People in wheelchairs are certainly not prevented from going shopping. However, if you plan to shop in a department store where you will need to use the elevators, it's a good idea not to shop at the busiest time of day. There is no sense in irritating many people who cannot help thinking that several people could have gotten on the elevator if you weren't taking up so much space.

I would not suggest that you ride the escalators. You are probably thinking, "Well, of course not, how ridiculous!" You may not believe it but I know a man who *does* ride his wheelchair on the escalator. Needless to say, he's very strong, daring, and unusual.

As far as the actual shopping is concerned, there is really no difference from that of a normal person. In fact, you have the advantage of a lap for carrying packages. The only hindrance is that sometimes aisles are narrow and partially stacked with merchandise. That means finding another route to the particular counter you want to reach.

One thing that is different for the wheelchair shopper is his range of vision. While "walking people" may overlook items that are placed on low shelves, it is those that are put up high that we might not see well (and get a stiff neck trying to, I can tell you!)

People in wheelchairs find it difficult to try on clothes in the store. It is better to pick out the clothes you like, try them on at home and return them if they are not suitable.

Although this chapter is about your relationship with the outside world, I will include here a bit about armchair shopping. When you shop by mail or phone, you avoid tiring yourself from hectic wheeling around from counter to counter, battling crowds and traffic. You select what you want from the many mail-order catalogues available and then either phone or write your order in. Often the ads in a magazine or newspaper for one of these companies will invite you to send in for a free catalog. If you have several mail-order catalogues to choose from, that's like going from store to store without actually doing it. Trading stamp catalogues can be a similar help. Some department stores accept mail or phone orders and state this right in their newspaper ads. For those who enjoy shopping, this manner of buying things is not very satisfactory. I, myself, have never cared for shopping and am quite content to do about three-fourths of it at home. I phone my orders in and my husband picks them up for me. He also returns them whenever necessary. It is really the easiest way to buy clothes for yourself.

Another way of easy shopping is the kind you do from the door-to-door salespeople such as Avon and other cosmetic firms or the Fuller Brush Company. This provides an opportunity to get toothbrushes, lipstick and make-up or household products like floor polish, brooms or dusting spray. It also is a good source of gifts—fragrant soaps, fancy packages of bath powder or shaving lotion for men.

Suppose instead of a morning of shopping you want to attend church. Church aisles are usually wide enough so that during a regular service you can sit in the aisle next to the pew where the rest of your family is sitting. However, if there is to be a processional up the aisle, such as the choir, you can stay in the back of the church until everyone is seated and then wheel to your spot. If the aisle is to be used at the end of the service, you should get out of the way before the service ends. You can go to the rear of the church before the end of a service in order to be out of the path of the people leaving. Of course, instead of sitting in the aisle, you can transfer to a pew, have someone move your chair out of the way, and get back into your chair later. Let me tell you, though, if you are accustomed to sitting on a cushion in your chair and leaning on the comparatively soft chair back, you will never believe how hard a church pew can be!

There are people in wheelchairs who wonder if it is possible for them to attend college. Up until fairly recently, they were prevented from furthering their education because they couldn't get around the buildings. Today, however, more and more schools across the country are taking steps to remove architectural barriers which hinder the handicapped. Some schools have done more than others along these lines. Basically, these school buildings have some or all of the following: ramps, in addition to stairs, extra-wide doorways, restrooms which can be used by the handicapped as well as the able-bodied, and telephones, water fountains and elevators accessible to those in wheelchairs. If you are interested in attending a school, inquire about the facilities available at the college of your choice. If there are schools in your vicinity, a trip to their campuses will be even more enlightening.

A list of the colleges which have made changes for the benefit of the handicapped can be obtained from the National Easter Seals Society.

Studying at home may be more practical or desirable for you. For a free list of accredited home study schools, write to the National Home Study Council.

I cannot be very specific on the subject of working from a wheelchair because there are so many different types of jobs. Obviously, some are difficult or even impossible for a wheelchair worker to perform. There are others that are very adaptable to working in a constantly sitting-down position, and still others which are more easily performed by a person who can stand and walk a little, possibly with braces and crutches.

For someone whose former job may now be impossible, there are additional problems. What can you do now? What new skills can you learn or are you interested in acquiring? One thing you can do is contact your local Division of Vocational Rehabilitation for information. They will assist you with training and transportation problems. Also, check with your local Goodwill Industries, where there is often vocational counseling and job training opportunities. What they have in each area varies so you will need to inquire.

In general terms, for working in a wheelchair you have to consider four things: (1) do you have the energy to stay on a job all day or even part of a day; (2) do you have transportation back and forth to work; (3) can you maneuver in and out of the areas in which you would have to work; and (4) is all the equipment you'd be working with accessible to you? Let us consider each of these separately.

Anyone who cannot answer "yes" to the question "Do you have the strength and energy to perform your job?" can forget about the other three points. For those who can hold up well for the necessary length of time, let us see what else there is to think about.

Naturally, transportation to and from work is of utmost importance. If you are able to drive a car with hand controls, and can get yourself and your wheelchair in and out of the car and the building, you can take care of this matter yourself. If not, perhaps you have someone willing to be your driver. Will that driver also be able to help you in and out of the building? Or will there be someone on the premises who will be willing to assist you each day? I want to mention here that some buildings which have a troublesome front entrance may have a more convenient one in back. Assuming we have gotten you into the building, I will go on to the third point.

Can you get around easily in all areas where you will have to work? If work includes going to different floors, is there an elevator you can use? If there is a self-operated elevator, can you manage it by yourself? Can you use the rest room? All these things will have to be thought about and discussed with your future employer. Sometimes, an impossible situation can be made possible by some simple alteration. An employer who is willing to hire a handicapped worker is generally ready to provide assistance when and where it is needed.

Even if you can get into the building and all necessary sections of it, you are still in bad shape if you cannot reach your equipment. However, changes will not necessarily have to be complicated. For instance, in an office, the size of filing cabinets can make a big difference. Two-drawer cabinets can be used from a wheelchair, whereas unless you are able to stand, the top of a four-drawer cabinet is unreachable. Then there is material kept in closets. Keep those things you most often use on a lower shelf. Less frequently needed articles can be obtained from an upper shelf by a co-worker.

36

Being in a wheelchair certainly does not prevent a person from voting. From a chair, though, you cannot reach the upper levers of the voting machine, especially not the one that closes the curtain. Anyone you wish can come in the booth with you and push the levers for the candidates you select. If you do not want to say the names out loud, you can write them down ahead of time and hand the paper to the person assisting you. Once, as I was leaving the building where I voted, I saw a man in a wheelchair and stopped to talk to him. He was carrying a walker with him and intended to use it to stand up in the booth. If you are able to stand, you may prefer to vote by yourself.

In most cities, there are groups for the handicapped which you can join. If interested, you might ask your doctor or physical therapist, if you have one, if he knows of any. There are often groups for specific illnesses such as cerebral palsy or arthritis—I belong, for example, to one for multiple sclerosis. There are also groups for the handicapped in general. One such group is the Indoor Sports Club, a national organization with chapters in various parts of the country. For information, write to their national newspaper, *National Hookup*.

A good group to get into with nonhandicapped people is one which deals with the architectural barriers in buildings. It's not just old buildings that are poorly equipped for the use of the handicapped, but often modern ones as well. Multiple stairs, inconvenient rear doors by which a wheelchair must enter, going through the furnace room, using the freight elevator and all sorts of out-of-way and undesirable sections of a building is common for the wheelchair user. If you have the opportunity to help prevent or eliminate some of these obstacles, I hope you will consider taking it.

It is easy for someone in a wheelchair to go to a restaurant. There are plenty of eating establishments that are not hard to get in and out of so there is no difficulty avoiding those places that have an abundance of stairs both at the entrance and inside. If in doubt as to the layout of a restaurant, call and inquire about it before going out.

When you go to a place to eat and are ready to get settled, the waitress will remove one of the chairs at the table so you can sit there in your wheelchair. If the table is especially low, it is advantageous to have desk arms on your chair. You can never get close to the table with a standard arm. Once when I sat at a particularly low and narrow table, I was glad to have removable legs on my chair so I could take them off and place my feet on the floor.

Movies and plays are also no problem to attend. There are just a few things to remember. Some theaters have a section where those in wheelchairs can sit without being in anyone's way. The theater isn't one of the places to be sitting in the aisle, although some may consent to that if you are in the last row. It is really best to transfer to an aisle seat and have a person who is with you roll your chair off to some out-of-the-way spot to be retrieved when you are ready to leave.

When requesting reserved seat tickets, specify that you are in a wheelchair and must have an aisle seat.

At public gatherings such as in auditoriums and sports arenas, people in wheelchairs generally get the best "seat" in the house—right up in front. These places ordinarily have elevated rows so it wouldn't be possible to sit anywhere except on the main floor with a wheelchair. Again, when ordering tickets for a reserved show, be sure to tell the ticket seller that you are in a wheelchair.

Unfortunately, the wheelchair user is not always treated kindly when it comes to public seating. There are places and occasions when you will be placed in the worst viewing spot available, and it is not unusual for someone in a chair to have to sit separately from the other people. I don't know what to do about it except complain, but in case you were not aware of this problem, I wanted to let you know.

Never having been athletic, I do not mind the necessity now of concentrating on sideline activities. Still, those who have been used to an active life in their earlier years do not have to sit in a corner and mope. A person who participates as much as he is able is bound to be happier and more likable. Naturally, some things such as skiing, skating, and biking have to be given up, but there are other activities. In fairly large cities, there sometimes are wheelchair basketball games, bowling teams and the like. You will have to inquire around your town what is available in your particular area. Anyone interested in organizing wheelchair sports should write for information to the National Wheelchair Athletic Association.

Swimming is something that many of the handicapped enjoy. A pool is often part of the equipment at veteran's hospitals and rehabilitation centers. Even a person who doesn't have full use of his arms can often hang onto an inner tube. Please do swim in a pool or lake where there is a lifeguard. At a pool, you most likely will need assistance to get from the chair to the edge of the pool and from there can get into the water yourself. When I swim, the only thing that bothers me is that when I tire of swimming, I cannot stand up in the shallow water. All I can do is hang onto a rail at the side of the pool and this is rather tiring. The pool we go to is made especially for the handicapped and has steps at the side on which to sit. Trouble is, my balance is so poor that I spend most of my time falling over. At a beach, this can be solved by placing a lawn chair in the water near the shore. When you tire of swimming and want to rest, you can get into the chair either by yourself or with some assistance, sit until rested, then swim again. Obviously it is not as easy to push a wheelchair over the sand as it is on your front sidewalk. You can engage a "muscle man" for this project or such a person can park your chair on more level ground and carry you to the water. My husband has found that it is a little easier to transport a wheelchair over a beach if you pull it backwards. He gets me as close as possible to the water, locks my chair, and carries me the remaining few feet.

There is no reason why a person in a wheelchair cannot go fishing. I've seen them fishing from docks and it can be done from a boat, too. If you are like me, you will never be able to sit on a backless seat, but nowadays that can be remedied. You can get boat seats of several different types —some made of fiberglass, some with padded seats, some with arms and some without—and there are also those that swivel. Many of them are collapsible for easy transporting in the car. They can be found many places—department stores, large mail-order catalogues, even trading stamp stores.

Obviously, you will have to have one or more assistants on your fishing trip. The ground leading to a lake or river

40

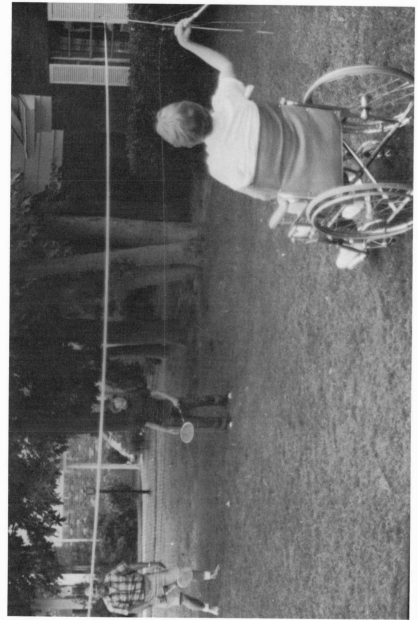

Playing badminton in a wheelchair.

is usually quite bumpy and it requires muscle power to get someone in a wheelchair over such territory.

If you are in a wheelchair, you cannot very well go on hikes through the woods when you go on a picnic, at least not at the average place. There are, however, parks that have trails especially designed for those in chairs. And volleyball with one or more people is possible. Although you cannot be as active as those around you, you can still enjoy being outdoors. From a vantage point, you can keep an eye on children. You can read, sew, write letters or work at some hobby (these are also perfect reasons for having a lapboard along), and still appreciate the scenery and breathe the fresh air. You certainly can participate when it comes time to eat and, again, a lapboard will be most helpful at such a time. See the chapter on aids for more about this useful item.

One of the biggest difficulties for the wheelchair picnicker is the inability to use public restrooms. If your parking spot has some privacy, someone can help you use a camper's toilet or bedpan in the car. Many people in wheelchairs have bladder problems and either have a catheter or must wear pants of some sort. Draining a catheter or changing to fresh pants can also be taken care of in the car.

You can bowl in a wheelchair at any alley but some places are much easier to move around in than others. Some have narrow, steep steps leading down to the playing area. It is a good idea to call ahead of time at the alley of your choice and find out what kind of setup it has.

If you haven't yet tried bowling from a chair, let me warn you not to expect too much of your first attempts.

You really need to practice a while before you get the feel of it. What you do is park at the foul line and lock your chair. Then, hanging on with one hand, you lean over as far as you can and roll your ball. Some alleys have a portable ramp that you can use to get up to the playing area when it's your time to bowl. If not, someone will have to get you up the step. When the place isn't crowded, they can let you use two alleys. When we go, my husband uses one and I stay permanently at the foul line of the alley next to him. He brings my ball to me each time. I find it best to situate myself on the left of the alley with my chair turned a little to the right.

You can get exercise right in your backyard by playing badminton or at least batting a birdie around. What you need is a partner who will fairly consistently hit the thing within your range. It helps to have one or two kids around who like to retrieve the ones you miss.

All sorts of hobbies can be enjoyed alone at home or with others at hobby or community centers. These include arts and crafts such as ceramics, painting and leatherwork, building models such as airplanes or automobiles and any type of collection. There are also many types of needlework—embroidery, knitting and crocheting, for instance. These are all sitting-down activities which, of course, are made for people like us. Check at your nearest community or hobby center if interested.

When it comes to sightseeing, there are many attractions open to the public all across the country which can be enjoyed by the handicapped. Some of these can even be seen from a car. Many of the buildings with historical features have only one or two small steps to overcome at the entrance and some have elevators inside. On the other hand, there are some places which are quite impractical, if not impossible, to get around in with a wheelchair. The best thing to do is ask about the facilities before venturing forth. As for national spots, you can learn what is available by reading *Guide to the National Parks and Monuments for Handicapped Tourists* by the President's Committee on Employment for the Handicapped.

Two thoughts about staying in a motel. If you make reservations for one on the phone, be sure to tell them that you are in a wheelchair and, unless the building has an elevator, you must have a first floor room. Also, many motels have miniature bathrooms. Then again, some of them have wide doorways and are roomy enough for a chair. This can be something else you will want to ask about.

For more specific information pertinent to the handicapped traveler, you may want to obtain a copy of *The Wheelchair Traveler*, a directory which is often updated. It lists hotels, motels, restaurants and sightseeing attractions from all over the U.S. that are particularly usable by the handicapped traveler. Besides names and addresses of these places, the directory includes door sizes, whether or not there are steps and a general rating system of usability.

3

HOUSEHOLD ARRANGEMENTS

In my opinion, if you can afford to make extensive alterations to a home to make it better for a wheelchair user, you
could hire someone to do everything and wouldn't need all
those changes anyway. Then, too, a lot of people today
move around the country fairly often and would find it
difficult to sell a house that was too different from the
ordinary. Still another group lives in rented houses or
apartments and would not be permitted to add to and
subtract from the home they live in. It would make more
sense, therefore, for the majority of the handicapped to
figure out how to make the most of what they have to work
with and decide what changes they need the most.

Since moving is hardly what you would call fun, if you
can get along well enough in your home, you don't need
to consider moving. There is quite a difference in homes,
though, and some are more adaptable than others for use

by someone in a wheelchair. Also, many homes require only a small amount of change to accommodate a wheelchair.

For instance, two of the homes I have lived in would have been quite adequate for my chair, I believe. In both of them, which we owned, I would have had no trouble getting into the bedroom from the hallway, and the bathrooms were large enough for me. The only alterations we would have needed for sure were an enlarged bathroom doorway, a handrail at the toilet, and a grab bar at the tub. If I had wanted to get outside by myself in either house, it would have been simple to build a ramp at either entrance.

I was not so lucky with the home we were living in when I first began life in a wheelchair. Building a ramp at the entrance would not have been a problem. We also could have easily put one leading out to the large storeroom, one step down from the kitchen, which was my laundry area. It was the larger flaws of this house that concerned us. For instance, the kitchen and living room were the only rooms I could get into by myself. Our narrow hallway was wide enough for my chair but there wasn't enough space to turn a chair into any of the bedrooms. That would automatically have meant dependence on others. Then there was the bathroom. It required a magnifying glass to find—hard enough for a person to walk, let alone wheel, into. This, actually, was the worst problem because there was no room to expand. Finally, in the two rooms I could manage to get into alone, the windows were so high that, even in my pre-wheelchair days, I had to stand on tiptoe to see out of them. That

46

meant that I couldn't keep an eye on my children when they were outside. This might sound like a minor point but it wasn't to me.

If you find yourself in a house that makes life intolerable for you, it might be a good idea to look over other homes. Possibly you can find another which will not be much different in price, to buy or rent, but will provide a much more liveable setup.

Instead of looking at other existing houses when we realized that a move was necessary, we built a new one. It was not a completely custom-built house. We took a floor plan used in a number of houses in the same area and made alterations on it. Mistakes were made in building this house but this is something that everyone who builds seems to experience. Now that I have lived in this house for a while, however, I would like to give my opinion of what are the most necessary and helpful features in a house where there is a person in a wheelchair.

Wide doorways make it a lot easier to move in and out of rooms with a wheelchair but you can do without them. When going through an especially narrow doorway, you can keep your fingers from getting smashed by pulling on the door frame with both hands to get through rather than keeping your hands on your wheels. If you do enlarge a doorway, you will find that a width of thirty-six inches is perfect.

The only doorway you might *have* to alter is the one to the bathroom. In modern homes, they are generally too narrow for a wheelchair to pass through. It is possible that even if you live in a rented home, the landlord will permit you to enlarge the bathroom doorway. After all, when you

47

have moved out, why should the new tenants object to a wider doorway?

For a long time I couldn't figure out why bathroom doorways are narrower than any other. Then someone told me what he thought was the reason and it sounds so logical I wonder why I never thought of it before. The bathroom is the only room in the house which has no furniture brought in or taken out of it.

Since bedrooms are usually reached from a hallway, it is important that there is turning space to get into them with a chair. Halls vary in width, and the arrangement of the rooms has much to do with how well you can enter them. If you are enlarging a hallway or building a new house to accommodate a wheelchair, I recommend that the hall be forty-eight inches wide. You may, however, want a builder to observe your attempts to turn and help you decide the width.

If you don't anticipate going out by yourself, ramped entrances are not vital. With someone assisting you, one or two steps are not a big obstacle. Both our entrances are ramped, but I never use the front one so they could have put steps there.

For those who live in a rented home or expect to be moving soon or often, a portable ramp may be the answer. This is practical where there is only one or two steps to manage because anything more would probably require too large of a ramp. You can ask at a lumber company if it is practical or possible and, if so, the best type of materials to use—just give them the details about your steps. Ramps are also available through your local medical supply companies or rental services.

(One comment here—when I say "you" can do this or that, I do not necessarily mean you, all by yourself. It can be you, along with a driver, doing something together, or someone else running an errand for you.)

Going up a ramp takes strength for the person in a wheelchair. I am often reminded of this when scaling the one leading up to our kitchen door from the carport. Without muscles, I would never make it.

To get off and on a porch without ramps or help, a Wheel-O-Vator can be put to use. This is an elevator designed to fit any porch with a patch of flat ground beside it. It only needs to be uncrated, set down, and plugged in. For more information, contact your local wheelchair dealer, limb and brace shop or rental agency. (Remember that not all places carry the same equipment.) The Wheel-O-Vator is manufactured by Wheelchair Elevators, Inc.

What people in wheelchairs need the most in a house is something that's hard to come by—floor space. Those high shelves in the kitchen and on the top of clothes closets and large attics are fine for other people but we need things down near the floor. If you have a large home, you have an advantage. With space, you can put shelves, cupboards, and other storage facilities wherever they are needed. You can place nearly everything where you can get your hands on it.

Metal shelving is really great. You can set up shelves in any width and height you desire. Also, unlike shelves that are secured to the wall, they can be moved around if you decide to move the furniture.

To me, the most important room to have done correctly is the bathroom. We made a huge mistake in ours by having

Toilet handrail, tub grab bar, and elevated toilet seat.

the bathtub arranged so that I can only approach it in a forward position. We should have allowed chair space next to the tub since I have removable arms on my chair and am quite expert at transferring sideways. Not only that, but I cannot even get close enough to the tub to clean it.

If you are going to have a new bathroom built or an older one remodeled, please be sure there is enough space for you to use the washbowl, toilet, and bathtub and to transfer in the way you can do it best. Have the person who is going to plan the room measure your chair (remember, they are not all the same size) and allow for turning space too.

A big help in transferring into the bathtub is a grab bar attached to the wall the tub sits against. The most useful handrail, though, is the one next to the toilet. Check with rehabilitation equipment establishments for the various types of both these rails. The Cleo Living Aids catalog shows several.

I didn't care for the toilet handrails I had seen at the time we built our house, so our builder instructed his workers to make me one. It's a dandy and will probably still be standing after the house falls down. It is made of a heavy metal bar about one-and-a-half inches wide and has a two-inch piece of railing over the top, which creates an indentation for a hand grip. Twenty-eight inches high, it is bolted to the wall and the floor. Now this is a single bar, which is ideal when you transfer sideways. Most of the ones I've seen sold commercially consist of bars on both sides of the toilet.

In the first chapter I talked about the elevated toilet seats which can be attached to a regular one. There is a more

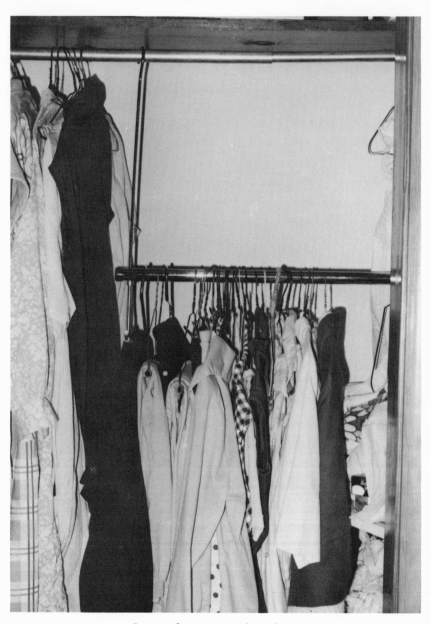

Lowered extension closet bar.

permanent way of handling this—the whole toilet can be raised and set on a block of wood. That evens things up better but it is not very attractive, although you can paint the wood white. Our builder again took care of this. His men cut plywood into circular shape the size of the toilet, glued the pieces together until it was three inches thick and covered it with white Formica. This was put between the top of the toilet and the seat, using seat bolts with extensions on them. With this, of course, you cannot use a toilet seat lid.

I would like to say something about linen closets. If I were to build our house anew, I certainly would plan a different cupboard for housing towels, sheets and the like. A tall, narrow closet, such as linen closets generally are, is very impractical and can cause much frustration. It is better to have a low, wide cupboard. If you do have a regular closet, it makes sense to put seldom-needed items on the upper shelves and the everyday ones on the lower. Also, if you have a situation such as we had, I recommend that you remedy it the way we did. Our linen closet had a door which only opened straight out and when my chair hit it, that was as far as I could go. I had a terrible time trying to reach anything inside. Finally we took the door off, and now there is no battle to go through just to get a clean towel. You can leave the shelves open if you want to or replace the wooden door with a vinyl closing. Sears and Montgomery Ward carry a wide variety of such doors.

We have two bathrooms but a linen closet only in the main one, so we had two wheelchair-level shelves put up in our closet to take care of the needs of our bedroom and attached bath.

A real help in the closet for wheelchair users is an extension bar that attaches to the regular closet bar and can be adjusted to the most convenient height for your use. This is the same kind you can hang in children's closets so they can put up and take down their own clothes. Extension bars can be bought wherever closet equipment is found.

If you are in a permanent home (that means you don't plan on moving soon), you might be interested in having someone make built-in dressers and chests for your bedroom. They can all be made at a low level and built to the floor so you will no longer have to clean under them. Of course, the furniture will always remain in the same place and rearranging will be quite limited.

The built-in idea can be carried over into the living room, too, for bookcases, stereo sets, and record cabinets. The same advantages and disadvantages as for the bedroom will prevail.

The most beneficial alteration in the kitchen will be the one made to the sink. Working sideways to peel potatoes, wash dishes, or even rinse them to put in the dishwasher, or, in fact, to do *anything*, is extremely awkward. I know because, at this writing, that's the way I must do everything. It will be worth your while and your money to have someone fix it so you can approach it in a forward position. The person who does this job will have to measure your chair and determine just what changes will need to be made. All cabinets under sinks are not exactly alike; neither are all wheelchairs, as I have already mentioned. The plumbing may be an obstacle, especially if you have a garbage disposal in the way.

Ideally, a person in a wheelchair should have a working

area completely clear underneath for the legs, enabling him or her to work in a forward position. If this surface is lower, it relieves fatigue on the arms. Such a setup needs to be built into the kitchen. A builder can make counter tops with openings under them, or put in a drop-in cooking top so you can cook facing the stove, and a wall oven can be included. The thing is, any arrangement is possible if you want to pay the price. Financing for such projects is sometimes available through your state's Division of Vocational Rehabilitation and the Federal Department of Housing and Urban Development (HUD), if it means that the homemaker will be independent after the changes. Investigate such possibilities with these two agencies.

As I said before, though, there are many people who cannot afford or are unable or unwilling to change over their entire kitchen. It may be far more practical to discuss how to make the best use of existing situations or in what way meal preparation can be simplified for the handicapped. This I attempt to do in the chapter on meal preparation.

In the kitchen, my cabinets are arranged as in any normal home. Things in front of the bottom shelves of the upper cabinets are within my reach and utensils I don't use constantly are kept on higher shelves and in the back of the bottom shelves. For the latter, I just have to anticipate my needs ahead of time and ask my husband or oldest girl to get them down for me.

My pots and pans are kept in a bottom cabinet as in any kitchen. To keep your most used pots and pans handy, you can attach a disappearing pan rack to the top of a cabinet, which pulls out in front of the cabinet when the door is open, and slides easily back in place. The rack has large hooks on which to hang the pots. Knape and Vogt Manufacturing Company makes such a rack. Your local hardware store may stock it.

Some people like to make use of pegboards attached to the inside of cabinet doors or the wall space under upper cabinets. Using the latter, frequently used items are out in the open and never need to be hunted for. Others find it convenient to have upright dividers built into a kitchen drawer so that some thin utensils such as cookie sheets, cake racks, and cupcake tins can be filed like office equipment. In some housewares departments, you can find a metal holder for the same purpose.

The only way my kitchen arrangement is a bit unusual is in where I have everyday dishes stored. Visitors seeking dishes to help set the table or looking for a glass or coffee cup are puzzled when they find none in the top cupboards. My everyday dishes are in a lower three-shelved cabinet, the most logical place for things that will be taken in and out constantly from a sitting-down position. For the first six months we lived in our house, I struggled to get out the cups from the back of these shelves. Then I got one of those large turntables (by Rubbermaid, available almost everywhere) and now, at the spin of a wheel, glasses, coffee cups, measuring cups and dessert dishes are always in front.

Besides dishes, you need to be able to put your hand on canned and packaged foods, spices, and other items. We were lucky to have a hall clothes closet we did not need so we had shelves put in it and made it a food closet. Now I can reach three shelves completely and the front row of the fourth. As in my dish cupboard, I keep within my reach the foods I will need often. The other things are on a higher shelf for my husband or children to get down for me. Several single and double turntables keep spices, puddings, soups and other canned goods at my fingertips and I thus avoid knocking down two or three cans or bottles every time I reach for something.

In my refrigerator, I've also got a turntable—one that came with five clear plastic pie-shaped containers, with lids, for leftovers. (That is, they are shaped like a slice of pie but are about three inches high). No longer do I find a plastic box of food in the back of a shelf three weeks after I put it in the refrigerator. Just a push with my fingers reveals what is on hand that needs to be finished. I have seen similar sets in the housewares sections of department stores but you can make such a setup by using any kind of turntable and plastic food storage boxes.

One of the handiest items in my kitchen is a pull-out board in the cabinet to the right of the stove. It is Formica-topped so I can take hot pans right off the burner and set them on the board. Best of all, I can work with everything in front of me rather than sideways.

Until I learned to use this board to scoop cake batter out of the large mixer bowl into a cake pan, I thought I was going to drop everything on the floor. A bowl, especially a heavy one, is quite awkward to dish out of in a sitting position. Now I push the cake pan on my board right up against the cabinet, rest the bowl on its side on the countertop and scoop it out. The edge of the counter gets somewhat messy, but that is a lot easier to clean up than batter spilled on the floor and maybe a broken bowl too.

A large board like this is an ideal place on which to use

an electric skillet because you can work in a forward position. Of course, it has to be large enough for the pan to fit on. There is one disadvantage, though, and it is the reason I never use my board for this—cooking this way means that the pan is jutting out in the room and not in a safe spot on a counter. Unless you are going to sit there and keep your eye on whatever is cooking, this can present a dangerous situation. It can be disastrous for a home with small children and equally so if, like me, you have a tendency to back up without looking.

A word about carpets. You probably already know that it takes a little more effort to wheel on a carpet than a bare floor and that your chair wheels leave marks on some materials. Anyone who uses crutches or a walker, in addition to a wheelchair, is sure to find that carpeting slows down his progress. We have no carpets in our home at all. Of course, if you have fairly new floor coverings, you will probably want to keep them in spite of the nuisance they create.

Throw rugs, on the other hand, are not only troublesome but dangerous for people using crutches or canes. They are good only for tripping over. They halt everything for those in wheelchairs, too. The only rooms where you can safely have them are those you will not need to go into.

4

AIDS

What housekeeping you can do on your own depends, naturally, upon your physical abilities. Perhaps you have very limited capabilities and can only take over a small portion of work. I guarantee that it will do a great deal for your morale if you can do anything on your own, however little it is. As far as answering the question: just what kind of work can be done from a wheelchair? The answer is: anything you can reach. Since there are some things that you can't reach, and some which, even though you can, are difficult and tiring to do, some chores must be done by others. Once you have accepted this fact, you need only decide what these tasks are and to whom they will be given. Your assistant could be your husband, mother, children, sister, friend or cleaning woman.

It is hard to say just how much I, myself, am able to do since my physical condition has, at times, been quite good and, at others, quite terrible. I have jumped from the inability to do anything at all to doing almost everything reachable and then back to very limited activity around the house. Since my energy is so come-and-go, I just do as much as I can when I can and put my children and husband to work at the other times.

It really doesn't hurt children to work around the house at an earlier age than most of their playmates. More than likely you will want them to be taking on some responsibility anyway. My kids are not overjoyed with their tasks but I let them know that there are things I simply cannot do and that they will *have* to and that's that. They made such a fuss, at first, about having to change their sheets themselves. "It's too hard!" they wailed. "We're too little to do it!" I ignored their protests and supervised the job for two weeks. Now they know which day their bed is to be done and they automatically tend to it. To ease the washing situation, we do one bed a day—and with five beds—that comes out nicely.

It is amazing what even a three-year-old can do by himself. I know from experience that he can strip beds, help carry laundry to the washer, help empty the dishwasher and set the table if you use unbreakable dishes, empty wastebaskets into the garbage can, retrieve toys from under beds, dust (although rather crudely) low pieces of furniture, and bring such needed items as tissues and paper towels.

In addition to human aids, there are all sorts of gadgets which the handicapped can use. Many are available from an ordinary department store. Read your newspaper ads carefully and you will often see them.

A good source of gadgets are the catalogues which are advertised in the rear of many home and women's magazines, especially those sold in supermarkets. The ads are more numerous the closer it gets to Christmas. These catalogues can be obtained by a postcard request. If there are things advertised and no mention of catalogues, you can write and ask if they would send one. Usually, once you buy an item or two from one or more of these companies, you get on the mailing list of others and begin to receive more catalogues than you really care to get. However, I find that if you don't buy anything from them, they eventually stop mailing their literature to you. Some have better merchandise and prices than others. Most of these items are fairly inexpensive, though, so you can send for a few things to see how well they serve without putting out too much cash.

Some of the articles advertised in these catalogues that are helpful to the handicapped are a thirty-inch magnetic reacher, a sponge-type tub scrubber, a window washer (the handle of which expands to three feet) and a bakeware storage rack for upright filing. All the mail-order firms constantly change their line so it is not possible to say where any particular piece of equipment might be found. For the widest selection of useful items, look in a Miles Kimball catalog. Several other companies are Helen Gallagher-Foster House and Walter Drake.

In addition to handy gadgets, these catalogues have all sorts of gifts for which you can send. Since we cannot hop into a car and drive off to the shopping center as easily as some people can, it is a real advantage to be able to select gifts by mail.

Using a reacher to get something out of a cupboard.

People with creative minds and who are handy with tools can dream up many aids, probably better than what can be bought. A word of caution—it is a good idea to try an activity with normal equipment first and see how well it can be used as is or with slight alterations. It is easy to accumulate a houseful of helps that may not even be necessary.

One of the difficulties of a person in a wheelchair is the inability to reach many things. Sometimes this can be solved simply by asking someone to get them from high shelves *before* they are needed, which, of course, calls for planning ahead. A reacher may be the answer for many. Several types are available from rehabilitation supply houses, wheelchair dealers or some of the above-mentioned mail order firms. There are different varieties and lengths. One kind is a giant-sized tongs, magnetized for metal pick-ups. Keeping this reaching device in one central spot of the house works out all right if it isn't a nuisance to get for every situation. If the only place it is needed is in a food cupboard or a certain closet or cabinet, the reacher can be left somewhere inside the storage space to be used when necessary. When reaching to lower shelves or picking up something from the floor is not easy, a reacher very close by is needed. Cleo Living Aids has one that looks like a huge wooden shears and is about a foot and a half long. I often keep mine next to me on my chair to use whenever needed. Sometimes I keep it in a corner of the kitchen and it gets knocked over. My kids think it is amusing to say that their mother "can't reach her reacher."

When an extension to your arm is needed only occasionally and for short distances, ordinary kitchen tongs might suffice. I have an eleven-inch long one which stays in a desk drawer to retrieve the pen I'm forever dropping on the floor. This is good to use when something falls in the space between the stove and refrigerator or for picking up a button from the bottom of a dryer. If they are not too high up, cereal boxes or cake mixes can be brought down to you with this.

A very simple aid in the home is an ordinary wire clothes hanger bent out of shape like this:

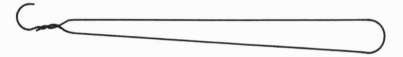

Figure 2. Clothes Hanger Bent Out of Shape

Before I acquired my reacher, I used the hanger for things like pulling down the towel and rag from the unreachable towel rack over the bathtub, straightening the drapes that had gotten folded up on the sofa top, closing hard-to-reach doors (the hook fits easily over the knob), and pulling jars or packages from the back of refrigerator or cupboard shelves to the front so they could be grasped. There are still situations which are solved better with the hanger than anything else. For instance, it's the best thing I have found for recovering my shoes, which are always getting shoved under the bed. This reacher can be even more useful if a magnet is attached to the end of it for picking up such items as pins and paper clips.

The one indispensable aid, in my opinion, is the lapboard, sometimes called a utility tray. These can be bought where wheelchairs and other rehabilitation equipment is

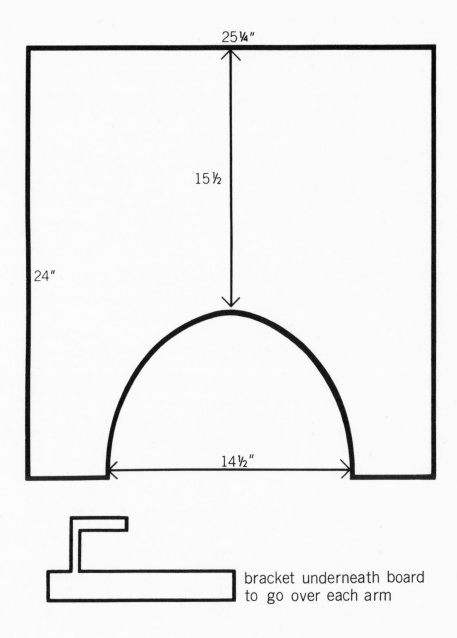

25¼"

15½

24"

14½"

bracket underneath board
to go over each arm

Figure 3. Lapboard

65

sold. A much larger and far more useful board than you can buy ready-made, however, is one you have custom-built for yourself. It is simple to make and not very expensive, but I consider it worth whatever it costs to have one made. I honestly could not get along without mine and nearly every day find a use for it. It can be made out of plywood and varnished or painted, and slides over the armrest of a chair with a bracket (see Figure 3). The measurements of mine are 25 ¼ inches across, 24 inches deep, 15½ inches from the peak of the cutout to the end of the board, and 14½ inches wide for the cutout. This cut can be made larger if you need more tummy room. The position of the arm bracket (mine is three inches long) is determined by the distance between the arms of your chair and the thickness of the bracket by the thickness of the armrest. Be sure you have the chair you will always be using when it comes time for someone to measure for the lapboard. All chairs are not the same size and all armrests are not the same either.

Although my board does not have one, it occurred to me that a Formica top would be great. Then you can take hot dishes out of the oven or pots off the burners and set them directly on the board. You can put down a cup of coffee without putting something under it to avoid marking the finish. Also, it is easy to clean. Now I'm hoping my board will wear out soon so I can get a new one made with a Formica top!

I'll be referring often to the lapboard in the pages to come. If you don't have one, you will probably think I bring up the subject far too often. Well, I do because it's so useful. The main thing the lapboard does is provide a ready table for you. This is especially helpful for those with a standard arm wheelchair, who have difficulty getting close to an ordinary table. It's a good place for writing letters, reading, and working on hobbies. If you don't have a desk and the kitchen table is set for a meal, you still have a clear spot on which to work. Also, anytime you need to carry something which would be likely to spill or is easily broken, the lapboard is much safer than your lap.

5

MEAL PREPARATION

If you have never tried cooking from a wheelchair, it is not something to jump into full force right from the beginning. It makes a lot more sense to try the easier things first and progress to the more difficult.

To me, the hardest part of a meal is actually its planning. When I first came home from a prolonged stay in the hospital, all I did was plan and supervise meals. My husband didn't mind following instructions like, "Now you turn down the oven to 250 degrees and set the timer for an hour," or "It's time to put the rolls into the oven," but if he had had to figure out what we would have for supper in the first place, he would not have appreciated that at all. So even if you are not able to do any cooking, you can still plan.

Let's talk about the necessary appliance for cooking—the stove. What you really need is one that has the buttons and dials in the front or the side and not at the top. With the latter, you not only can't reach but you *shouldn't* reach across the burners—it's dangerous. I advise you not to cook at all unless you have the right kind of stove.

Many stoves have the buttons on top, however, so suppose you have one and cannot, at this time, get a new one? For one thing, even if you have to let someone else do the top-of-the-stove cooking, that doesn't stop you from mixing together a salad, casserole or dessert. You can also make the coffee, set the table, and take the bread out of the freezer to thaw.

There are small appliances which can be substituted for a stove or be used in addition to one. An electric skillet is one which comes to mind. Using one eliminates the need for reaching across dangerously hot burners. When you are cooking bacon and eggs or pancakes for breakfast, the skillet can be used right at the table, thus avoiding the need to carry the food from the stove.

For stove cooking without using a stove, there is the one- or two-burner hot plate, sometimes called a buffet range, which can be set on a counter.

Wall ovens would be at chair level for getting hot dishes out of the oven. Of course, food removed from the oven will have to be put on a lapboard or table. It is much harder to lift dishes from ovens and broilers below the seat of your chair.

Small oven-broilers used on a counter top are much easier to manage than a regular oven. If you have a counter spot with open space underneath for your legs, getting food in and out is fairly simple. There are various types of these so, if you are interested in buying one, it would be wise to go to several department stores and look at them personally.

There are numerous ways to simplify meal preparation. One is to plan easy meals, especially in the beginning. The greatest boon to any cook is the casserole. It can be prepared early in the day for baking when the dinner time nears. There are many varieties to choose from, and it is also a good way to use up leftovers. The basic ingredients, of course, are some sort of meat, fish or eggs, and any number of vegetables mixed with a sauce. Usually there is some starchy food included—potatoes, rice, noodles or macaroni—and it is often topped with bread crumbs or cheese. Although some casseroles require the cooking of meat, there are many that do not. The meat can be ham, which only needs cutting up, canned corned beef or tuna fish. Cooking macaroni is not difficult, as I will explain, and neither is rice. I even have several recipes which call for uncooked rice. If you use canned vegetables, there are no vegetables to cook. There is no need to make a white sauce nowadays either. Just about everything tastes good when cooked with a sauce made from a can of any of the cream or cheese soups and a small amount of milk.

Before going on, let me say this in regard to assembling anything—whether a casserole, meatloaf, or dessert. If you will be using your hands to cut up, chop, form or whatever, don't forget to have on your working area a damp rag or some paper towels on which to wipe off your hands. It is irritating to get your hands messy and then have to wheel to the other side of the room for something with which to clean them. By then, you most likely have to wash off the handrims of your chair. In other words, think ahead.

Rejecting casseroles usually means the major part of the meal will be the meat. If you can lift the broiler pan out of the oven yourself or use a portable broiler-oven, all sorts of meat, from steak to hamburgers, can be cooked. Meatloaf can be fixed early in the day and popped into the oven when it is time to start supper. There is also nothing involved in heating fishsticks. And for an easy top-of-the-stove meat which requires no frying, there are always frankfurters.

Some types of potatoes—such as French fries or baked potatoes—need little preparation to use. Peeling potatoes can be more of an obstacle. For instance, peeling potatoes or anything else sideways at the sink is very uncomfortable. Try doing it at the kitchen table, then carrying the container of potatoes to the sink balanced on your lap or on a lapboard. You can also do the peeling directly on the board spread with a newspaper. If you have only one hand to work with, you can still peel potatoes. A peeler made of one or several nails thrust upward through a piece of wood does the trick. They can be bought where rehabilitation supplies are sold (Cleo Living Aids, for instance) or one can be made with wood and nonrusting nails. If interested, ask at a hardware store.

Most salads can be partially or completely prepared ahead of time. Ingredients such as vegetables and fruit can be sliced or chopped and put into the refrigerator to be combined later with salad dressing.

When the lid of the salad dressing jar is balky, you need an Easy Jar Opener, a V-shaped apparatus that attaches inconspicuously to the bottom of an upper cabinet. Using one hand, you can open everything, from nail polish to

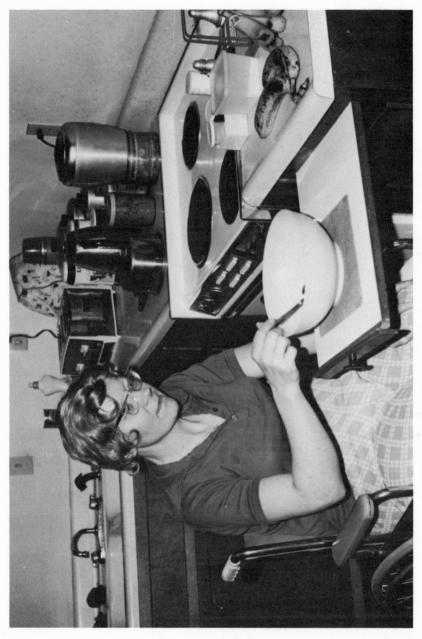

Mixing, using the sponge cloth spoken of in this chapter, and the pull-out board mentioned in Chapter 3.

quart-size jars. It is doubly useful for the person who must work one-handed because, with it, you can also close jars. Look for it in mail order catalogues.

There are so many different kinds of bread that need nothing done to them or require just a quick trip to the oven. There is a variety of refrigerated biscuits and brown-and-serve rolls, and then there is the bread you can get at the local bakery. All you have to do is decide which type to serve.

When you are used to cooking sitting down, you can take on something complicated with which to end a meal. Meanwhile, there are many desserts which are good but practically effortless to fix. There are, of course, frozen cakes and pies which you merely thaw out and serve, and ice cream, which you surely better not thaw out! From there you can go to instant pudding, which needs only a little arm work with an egg beater; gelatin desserts, which just need to be mixed with water; and cooked puddings, which need stirring for a few minutes at the stove. If you have a meatloaf and salad ingredients prepared, you can whip up one of your favorite pies. I used to avoid making pies, even though I love them, because I could never make a good crust. Now I buy frozen pie shells and concentrate my efforts on the fillings.

Preparing dessert often means the need for mixing bowls, which are often made of breakable glass. When full they are also heavy and awkward to lift from a seated position, especially if the task has to be accomplished with one hand. Stainless steel bowls are much lighter, and plastic even more so. There are two drawbacks to using plastic bowls, though. One is that they are so flexible you have to

74

be extra careful when pouring from them and the other is that their edge is no good for cracking raw eggs. If all bowls are difficult to handle, try mixing in a large pot. That way, when you mix, lift or pour, you have a handle to grasp.

An ordinary eggbeater requires two hands to operate. A one-handed model can be bought some places where rehabilitation equipment is sold. Another beating device meant to be used by one hand is the whisk, which is inexpensive, comes in various sizes and can be found in housewares departments.

To keep a bowl from dancing all over the table or counter while you mix something or ending up on the floor, the perfect solution is to set the bowl on a wet sponge cloth. Sponge cloths are sold in housewares departments of ordinary department stores or can be ordered through Fuller Brush. Looking like thick pieces of cloth but being sponges, they are stiff when dry. They are especially useful when you have only one usable hand. They really work.

Many dishes include eggs. The safest way to carry eggs from the refrigerator to the stove or table is by putting them in an empty egg carton which you have saved for the purpose and have resting on your lap. As for cleaning up a raw egg smashed on the floor, I cannot give you a number of ways to handle this because it happened to me only once. Some things I am glad to experiment with, but I guarantee that I'm not going to smash eggs all over my kitchen floor just so I can try different methods of cleaning them up! I would suggest using that oh-so-useful small mop I talk about in the chapters about housekeeping.

It really is not possible to keep an eye on pans set on the

back burners of the stove. They are too far back for you to look into unless you are very tall even when sitting down. You can see into these pans by holding a long-handled mirror over the top. Remember, though, if you have to throw in some vegetables or stir the ingredients, you will have to reach over the pots on the front burners. To avoid this, make sure someone is with you when you need to use that many burners or, if you know you will have no help at meal time, prepare something easy to handle, such as a casserole.

When something has finished cooking and needs to be set off a burner, sit on the side opposite it and pull the pan over to a cold burner. That way you are not holding your arm over a hot burner.

Pans filled with water can be quite heavy and, thus, difficult to get from the sink to the stove. If the kitchen is going to be remodeled, you can have a longer than normal spray hose put on the sink, one that will reach the stove for the purpose of filling pots. If you are able to lift a filled pan from the sink to the counter and have a stove on the same side of the room, you can slide the pan along the counter until you get to the stove. If your sink and stove are across from each other, possibly you can set the pan of water on your lap and then lift it to the stove. If you are afraid of spilling, you can use a lapboard. The pot can still be filled if lightweight containers can be lifted but not heavy ones. Several things, such as plastic cups or glasses, can be filled with water and set next to you on the chair, then carried to the stove and dumped out into the empty pot.

A pot of cooked food is not only heavy but hot. If it is soup, it can be ladled into bowls right at the stove and then carried to the table on a lapboard or pushed along on a utility table or serving cart. Vegetables could be scooped out of a hot water bath with a small sieve. When the difficulty is not with lifting the pan but in draining the food, dump the pan's contents into a colander set in the sink.

Pastas (spaghetti, macaroni or noodles) that have finished cooking need draining, of course, but it is usually in large, heavy pans which are no small feat to lift from a sitting-down position. The best way to handle this is to use a spaghetti cooker, sometimes called a food blancher. You'll find them wherever pots and pans are sold. This has an inner pan filled with holes. When your macaroni is cooked, you raise up the inner pan and the water drains into the outer one. Then you have a fairly lightweight container of drained macaroni, which you can put into a dish or slide to the sink to be rinsed. Someone else can empty the pan of water later.

Frying anything requires close watching and usually means turning the individual pieces of food. Working at the stove sideways is quite awkward but may be the only way for many to accomplish the job. As I have already said, cooking will be simpler if you have a dropped cooking top with space underneath for your legs or can use an electric skillet on a counter which is open under it, or at the kitchen or other type of table.

That is an idea you might think about if there is plenty of kitchen space—a small table with leg space under it on which to use such things as an electric skillet or portable oven while sitting in a forward position. Some type of table like the one meant for a portable sewing machine might be used.

Draining off grease when frying can be a major problem if you have to lift the heavy pan containing hot grease. You can take care of the matter easily by tilting the pan with one hand and drawing in the grease with a baster in the other, depositing the grease in a container set nearby. As is true of many useful gadgets, a baster can be bought in a housewares department. When there is only a small amount of grease to be removed, it can be done with paper towels.

Before a meal can be eaten, the table must be set. You can pile a whole tableful of dishes on the lapboard. As wonderful as the board is for so many activities, to me, it is a hindrance for this one. First of all, with the board on, it is difficult to reach for my dishes on a shelf below me. Secondly, when I get to the table with a board full of dishes, it is awkward to transfer everything to the table. Instead, I carry my dishes balanced on my lap with the silverware laying on the stack of dishes and keep glasses and cups beside me on the chair. In another trip, I get incidentals such as napkins, salt shakers and the like. If you do not feel that dishes are too safe with you when setting or clearing the table, you can avoid cleaning up broken dishes, and frequently having to buy new ones, by using a set of melamine dinnerware.

Getting a completed meal from the stove to the table can be accomplished several ways. Someone else can convey everything to the table. I like that idea. Since my husband is home most of the time for supper, I reserve this job for him. As I've said before, if you are able to lift a dish out of the oven by yourself, you can set it on a lapboard. People with loss of sensation in the hands should use oven mittens with asbestos palms. An older child can help lift heavy dishes. You can also set the food on a utility table, the kind made for kitchens with three shelves on it. A hostess cart, serving cart or portable TV stand would all serve the same purpose and many have handles to grip as you push them along in front or beside you.

Don't *ever* set a hot-from-the-oven dish or pan on your lap. Even if *you* might not feel it, your legs do, believe me.

As for the coffeepot—again there's the lapboard. Also, some people keep an electric pot plugged in at the table and avoid carrying it altogether.

Once your meal is finished, your table is loaded with dirty dishes and probably a few things like chicken bones, leftover vegetables and crumpled napkins. The normal woman puts leftovers in the proper containers, collects garbage in a dish, stacks the dishes and carries them to the sink, then wipes off the table with a dishrag, possibly sweeping the crumbs into her hand and dumping them into the sink or garbage dish. The wheelchair housewife cannot carry dishes or crumbs in her hand very easily. She needs at least one hand to wheel her chair. My answer to carrying anything is always one of these three: 1) somebody else, 2) lapboard, or 3) your lap. As in setting the table, you can stack quite a bit on a lapboard but you can't get close to the table with it on the chair. When you get to the sink, the board is again in the way. If no one else is around to help and you don't have or want to use a lapboard, that leaves your lap. Doing it this way requires a number of trips back and forth. Piling dishes too high on the lap can be disastrous. It doesn't take long, however, to determine how high is too high. Again, melamine dishes can be used rather than breakable ones. When I clear the table, the dishes set on my lap while the glasses and cups are beside me on the chair. I put all the silverware and any garbage in a small aluminum pan, wipe off the table, and sweep any remaining crumbs into the pan.

Scraping and rinsing dishes for washing is not what I call a comfortable task to have to do sideways. What you need is a sink where you can sit in a forward position. I hope you have one. Maybe I will sometime, but I do not at this writing.

The greatest way to take care of the necessary chore of dishwashing is with a dishwasher. Those of you who have one will undoubtedly agree with me.

Washing dishes by hand isn't really so bad if you can sit facing the sink with your legs underneath it. Sitting sideways at the sink is especially uncomfortable if you have cabinets and a countertop at right angles to the sink and cannot get next to it. If you can't get your sink altered, perhaps you can get someone else to do the dishes on a regular basis.

Using Teflon-coated pans eases the cleaning-up process. If the dirty ones are soaked before you eat, they are ready for a simple rinsing out later.

A person with loss of sensation in the hands should wear insulated gloves when washing dishes to help increase the grasp on things which slip easily and prevent hands from burning. To determine a safe water temperature, someone with normal sensation can put water in the sink as hot as he can stand it and then test it with a candy thermometer. Keeping in mind what that safe temperature is, the handicapped dishwasher can test his water in the same way when he has filled the sink for the job.

Here is an idea of how to wash dishes in a comfortable way, if you cannot use the sink. This method requires a lapboard and a spray hose. Put the dishpan with detergent in it in front of you on the board and fill the pan using the hose. Then take the dirty dishes, which have already been scraped or rinsed, from the sink or counter and wash them in the pan. Next, put the washed, soapy dishes in a dish-rack, spray them off with hot water from the hose, and leave the dishes to air dry.

My last word on dishwashing is—are you sure you can't get a dishwasher?

6

GENERAL
HOUSEKEEPING

When I first began my household duties from a wheel-chair, I did not have the slightest notion how to go about them. I learned how through trial and error, over many months, and continue to learn new techniques even now. In the hope that I can be of help to others in wheelchairs, I have set down here methods which I have used or that I know others use.

Of course, no one can tell you how you should approach each situation. What one person finds a satisfactory solution to a problem, another may find extremely awkward. Also, you will not find two people with exactly the same injury or illness, the same size family, children of the same age, and identical homes. You can only decide what is best for you by trying different ways of doing things. It helps a great deal though to have a basic pattern to follow when you start out.

To begin with, you should keep in mind that everything takes you longer than it does a normal person, even just plain getting out of bed! If others don't believe it, have someone try an experiment with you. A simple way of making this quite clear is to get something out of the refrigerator, say a jar of salad dressing and a package of baloney. The normal person: (1) opens the refrigerator door, (2) takes out the two items, (3) slams the door, (4) carries the items to the table, and (5) sets them down on the table. Nothing to it, right? Ah, but the person in a wheelchair has to: (1) open the refrigerator door, and as he does this, back up his chair to get out of the way of the door, (2) move in closer so he can reach the shelves, (3) get out the two things, (4) set them as securely as he can, either beside him on the chair or on his lap, (5) back up so he can close the refrigerator door, (6) close the door, (7) wheel to the table and, finally, (8) set the items down. This difference between those on foot and people on wheels never occurs to the average person. I have had several people to whom I've explained this say, "Why, that's right. I never thought of it."

In my initial housekeeping days, I attempted to follow a rigid schedule. Knowing that everything was going to take me longer, I tried to spread the work over six days with very specific duties for each day. On paper it looked great but in practice it was a complete failure. Everyone has to contend with the interruption of phone calls, salesmen at the door, or unexpected visitors. The mother of young children has the additional time-consuming tasks of wiping up spilled milk, cleaning up a child who has fallen in the mud, and settling fights. For the wheelchair housewife, these things can take large chunks out of a too-rigid schedule. It is far better to keep in mind the most important things to get done in any particular day and concentrate on them, doing others if there is time and energy.

The two rooms that always need the most attention are the living room—or the den, if that is used more—and the kitchen. You, and your family and visitors as well, will more than likely spend most of your time in one of these two places. It makes more sense then, when your time is limited, to straighten and dust the living room and to keep the kitchen floor mopped than to worry about the dust that has accumulated under your bed.

Try to be your own efficiency expert. Always ask yourself if there isn't a better way to do what you are doing or a more convenient place to keep supplies. This is very important to me. This disease I have, multiple sclerosis, has a weird pattern of energy and fatigue. Although I have strong arms, I tire very easily, some days more than others, so you had better believe that I do everything in the simplest and least exhausting method.

One thing you can do to alleviate housework somewhat is to alternate the heavier and more tiring tasks with a "sit still" activity. For instance, instead of going from one room to another with the vacuum cleaner, do one room and then stop to fold some clothes, make out your grocery list or prepare a gelatin dessert for supper. For that matter, your less active period doesn't need to be work. You could begin a letter to a friend or read some pages from a book or magazine. After a few minutes, you can move the vacuum cleaner to another room and work on it.

When I get to feeling really tired, the only thing that refreshes me to carry on my work is a rest on the bed. It's very logical why this does the trick. When a person has been on his feet for a while, he rests by sitting down. We are sitting all the time so the only break we get is when we lie down.

The majority of dusting jobs can be done the same way by the wheelchair worker as by the normal person. In fact, some things are even handier from a seated position. Out-of-reach furniture, window sills and cobwebs can be taken care of by: (1) someone else, (2) dusting attachment of the vacuum cleaner, (3) a dustmop, or (4) an old-fashioned feather duster, which can still be bought at housewares departments.

The most exhausting job done in the living room is vacuuming the sofa, yet this is something that needs to be done at intervals. If you find it as tiring as I do, you can improve the situation in several ways. First, there's that great method I am always talking about—keep this chore for someone else to do. Second, if you must do it yourself, lie down and rest for a few minutes afterwards. Third, there's a way to eliminate this job altogether and that is by having your furniture upholstered in vinyl. Then, all you need to do when it gets dirty is wash it off, usually with just a damp cloth and occasionally with soap and water.

The ideal piece of equipment for washing all around vinyl-upholstered furniture is a short handled mop with a small head. It has a handle a little longer than a toilet bowl brush, a head which could be wrung out with one hand, and can be used with one hand. Fuller Brush calls theirs a spatter mop, Stanley Home Products, a bathroom mop.

Some department stores also carry them. This is good, of course, for other things besides vinyl furniture. I have three of them myself in more than one room, so they don't have to be carried around. In future pages, you will see how many jobs can be handled well with this little mop.

To get back to removing dust, though—you can cut down on some of it by being selective in your purchasing. What I mean is, instead of buying a living room chair with a lot of wood portions, you can choose one that's all fabric-covered. Rather than an ornately carved table, you can pick one with simple lines. Also, there are table lamps without a lot of dust-catching nooks and crannies.

In the bedroom, what you can dust might very well be determined by the size of the room and what pieces of furniture you can reach by yourself. Even if you can take care of most of it, you may want someone else to do the dresser mirror or a hanging light fixture.

When it comes to cleaning a kitchen, the various spray-and-wipe-off cleaners seem as though they were made just for people in wheelchairs. Using them, there is no worry about transporting a cleaning mixture that may slosh on the floor while you carry it. You can keep the bottle (usually plastic, another recommendation for it) beside you on the chair and a damp sponge on your lap or a rag draped across your chair arm. Thus simply equipped, you can go about the kitchen wiping away fingerprints on woodwork or walls, the inevitable marks made by your footrest on appliances or juice stains on the kitchen table. These cleaners can also be used for counter tops, the stove, sink—anything washable.

Although these cleaners are very effective for the jobs I

mentioned, when you want to clean the entire front of the refrigerator or shine up the coffeepot, they give a streaky appearance. For such things, I like to use a small amount of rubbing alcohol on a paper towel. This is good for metal items that do not shed paint and I like the antiseptic smell.

There is a corner of my kitchen counter that I cannot reach. It is easiest, of course, to ask someone else to clean it for me. If you have a similar situation and want to handle it yourself, you can use the already mentioned little mop, possibly one that is specifically designated for use in the kitchen. Actually, the entire counter top can be washed with such a mop. If there are spots only a few inches too far away, a small dishmop works fine. They add about ten inches to your arm and can be bought at the dime store.

Oven cleaning is an ideal job—for someone else. If you insist on doing it yourself, let's see if we can make it a little easier for you. (I'm not so smart—I do mine by myself, too!) Obviously, a wall oven is much easier to clean than the conventional kind. It's at your level when you are in a sitting position. With a regular oven, this is normally a down-on-the-knees job, but this is, naturally, out for you or you wouldn't be in a wheelchair.

Here is a way to clean the oven. If there are a lot of crumbs in it, vacuum it out first. Then decide whether or not the racks, which are the hardest portion to do, need a cleaning this particular time. If not, remove them so that you can reach the rest of the oven. There are all sorts of oven cleaners, so use the one you prefer. Obviously, when it comes to wiping out the dirt, you need something beside your hand to reach all surfaces. That versatile small mop could be used for this purpose. Any long-handled device to which you could attach a rag might be tried also.

About those racks. Since I use a spray for which you need a warm oven, I spray the racks while they are in the oven. Then, after the required waiting period, I take them out and put them on my lapboard or the kitchen table, which I first cover with several thicknesses of newspaper. After cleaning out the oven, I can scrub off the racks with a wet rag and a pot scraper.

Since it can be reached from a wheelchair, the oven door can be done after the rest of the oven is cleaned or at another time. Most doors can be removed, too, by someone else and put on the table, where you could work on it in front of you.

The best solution to oven cleaning is to have a self-cleaning oven. If you are in the market for a new stove, do think of how great this would be, even though this type might cost more than the regular kind. I keep hoping mine will break down so I can get one of these but it will be just my luck that ours will still be doing fine fifty years from now. However, if I get rich, I might just buy one anyway!

A friend of mine hates to clean the bathroom while I would rather do ten bathrooms than tackle the kitchen. Regardless of your sentiment about bathrooms, how can this job be done best?

The washbowl can be cleaned in an ordinary way. The tub is more of an obstacle. If you can get next to it and run some water with cleaning solution in it, you can wash the tub with a broom. This may sound crazy, but it works and keeps your broom clean at the same time. You can do this with a regular mop and the small one is great for it, too. Also, mail-order firms carry a sponge mop especially meant for washing the tub. Actually, though, if you always use bubble bath in the water and rinse it out well after a bath, a lot of scrubbing isn't even necessary.

In my own tub, every so often I clean the top of the tub, soap dish and the faucets in a way that's a little different. I keep an alcohol-saturated rag within my reach when I am in the tub myself. Then, when my bath is finished, I clean those parts of the tub that I cannot reach at any other time.

The spray-on type of cleaner works well on tile walls but the ones around a tub would be unreachable. Possibly you can do part of the tiles by hand and another person can do the other portions.

There is nothing difficult about using a toilet bowl cleaner but it is awkward to reach around the outside of a toilet to clean it. That little mop I've been talking about is good both for this and for cleaning the top of the baseboard.

Whether or not you can make up a bed by yourself depends on if you can get around it with your chair. If you have a large bedroom where you can ride around both sides of the bed, you can make it up with ease. If one side of the bed must be against the wall, difficulties arise. You can smooth the sheet and blanket under the pillow by using a yardstick or other long-handled device but I fail to see how you can remove soiled sheets and put on clean ones. In my house, I can only get at my own bed. My children do their own. Two of them sleep in bunk beds which would be impossible for me to make up anyway.

Washing windows is another excellent choice for the "let somebody else do it" list. I did very little of this myself even when I was able-bodied, so I'm certainly not going to start now. However, you can get a long-handled squeegee in a department store to use for this purpose, if you wish. A pail of water could be kept beside you on a dolly for easy transporting.

One thing I am pretty certain you will not find a way to do is to take down and put up curtains and drapes. So if you need someone to do that job, you might as well have them do the windows too. You can make the care of curtains a lot less work by using those made of such noniron-able materials such as permanent press and fiberglass. Candidates for washing them might be more willing if it is known that no ironing is involved.

Mirrors are generally placed too high for the wheelchair worker to clean. I sometimes clean off the bottom of a mirror on a medicine chest that has been splashed on but I cannot do the whole thing myself. This is a simple job for a child to do with a squirt can of window cleaner and a paper towel. That's how it most often gets done at my house.

Maybe watering plants sounds like something which could not possibly present problems. Well, normally a person fills a container with water, walks to where the plants are and waters them. However, when you're in a chair and need your hands to wheel to your destination, you have to consider how you will carry the water. One way to do it is in a pitcher or jar carried on a lapboard, although if you have only one or two plants, putting on the board for this is a nuisance. You can try carrying a glass of water beside you on the chair, possibly wedging something against it to keep it from toppling over. If you usually wear slacks, setting the glass between the thighs works fine. One caution: don't fill the container too high and take those door sills nice and easy. If you have a preschooler around the house, he will probably be quite willing to carry the glass for you. If you don't trust him with a glass, make it a plastic cup.

For an ivy or philodendron plant which hangs down above your head, I hope you are not as dumb as I am when it comes time to water it. I used to fill up a glass of water and then wonder, since I couldn't see over the top of the plant, if it was getting any water and how much. Finally, after I hate to tell you how long a time, it came to me that all I had to do was put just a small amount of water in the glass and then I would know.

For any kind of hand sewing or mending, I cannot imagine anything more convenient than the lapboard. Using it, things like scissors, needles and the like are right in front of you. Then, if the phone or doorbell rings, all those dangerous items that you don't want kids to get into are right under your watchful eye. Another advantage to using a lapboard for mending is that you can accomplish this chore while keeping an eye on a cooking pot. Parked right next to the stove, needle and thread working away, you can still stir the pudding occasionally or check to see if the pot roast needs any water added to it.

The board is also a help for those who are visually as well as physically handicapped. With the board on, you can lean close to your sewing without worrying about falling out of the chair. If the eye of the needle is too small to see, you can get a needle threader from a mail order firm. They are inexpensive and really do work.

When it comes to sewing machines, a portable set on a table, working the foot control by hand (also on the table)

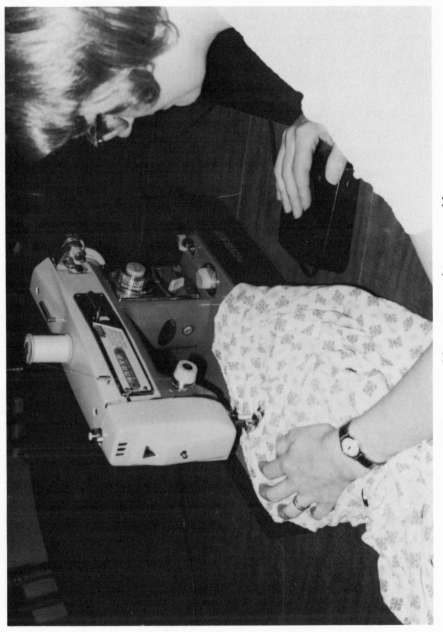

Using a portable sewing machine on a table, working the foot pedal by hand.

and guiding the material with the other hand, would seem to me to be the best for the wheelchair sewer. However, with a knee-control machine, if you cannot move the lever by knee, you can control it with one hand, again guiding the material with the other. It's a tight squeeze between the sewing machine legs for a wheelchair. You can get closer if you have removable legs on your chair and take them off. Another possibility is to transfer to a regular chair and use it at the machine.

7

FLOOR CARE

Since a good part of housekeeping involves sweeping, mopping, waxing or vacuuming floors, this subject deserves a chapter of its own.

We will start with the simplest form of floor care—sweeping. Some people like to work with a short-handled broom. Broom handles can be cut off halfway or at any desired length. I prefer a long handle, myself, because it requires less bending. Mine is a lightweight push broom which can be picked up with two fingers and is easily manipulated with one hand. It was bought at a Stanley party, but Fuller Brush has a similar type and a trip to your local department stores will reveal where else you can find one. Instead of a broom, some people find a dustmop better to work with. The only way to know what will work best for you is to try different methods. For instance, when you have worked with a long-handled broom first, you will know whether or not you want to shorten the handle.

If the front caster wheels on your wheelchair have spokes, the handle of a regular dustpan can be propped against them. However, for those who experience difficulty in bending, a long-handled dustpan is much better. They are not in abundance so it is a good idea, if you want to buy one, to check by phone as to their availability in your locality. I called two of the largest stores in my city to see if they carried long-handled dustpans. At one I was told that they did not, at another that they used to but don't anymore. I found one, though, at our local hardware store. That is a good place to ask for them. I say ask rather than look because even if you don't see one, they may be able to order one for you. These dustpans stand up on their own and have a handle which reaches higher than the arm of a wheelchair. My kids think they are great.

Now let's mop the floor. As always, equipment comes first. Again, as with a broom, try a regular mop before deciding if you want a long or short handle. The long-handled mop can be grasped with both hands when scrubbing stubborn spots. Unless you are very strong and can squeeze out and work with a heavy string mop, I would not consider using anything but a sponge mop. They are wrung out either by pushing two halves of a sponge head together with a lever, or by pushing down on the handle of a one-piece head.

When you have the kind of mop you want, you next have to consider the best way to wet it. If you are going to use a pail, it can be filled by means of a shampoo hose from the sink or bathtub or directly in the tub if you are able to lift a filled pail out of it. To move the pail around the house to the various rooms to be washed, it can be put on a dolly or lapboard, or placed on the floor and pushed along by your wheels (watch out for those door sills!) If you want to avoid transporting the pail, water can be run directly into the tub. The only disadvantage is that when water is in the tub and you are doing the kitchen, you have to make frequent trips back and forth. How do you carry a wet mop? Put something on your lap to protect your clothes, such as several thicknesses of newspaper or a piece of plastic sheeting or bag, and set the mop on top, resting the handle on your shoulder.

For once-over-lightly jobs in the kitchen with a damp mop, the simplest thing to do is wet the mop at the sink, which can be scrubbed out with cleanser afterward.

Before washing the kitchen, you will want to get the chairs off the floor. You cannot pick them up and carry them to the next room while moving in a wheelchair. You can put them in front of your chair and shove them along, or just move them enough out of the way so that you can wash a small patch of floor and then return them when the floor dries. If the chairs are not too heavy to lift, you can turn them upside down on the table while you do the floor, as is done in restaurants.

Sometimes, especially when mud and grass have been tracked in from outside, it looks as though you will have to mop a floor even though you just did that job two days earlier. I find that, often after I sweep or vacuum that floor, it doesn't look nearly so bad. You can then treat the worst spots with a damp mop.

For wiping up spills and small spots, the perfect thing to use is, again, that short-handled mop referred to in the chapter on general housekeeping. If the floor you are going

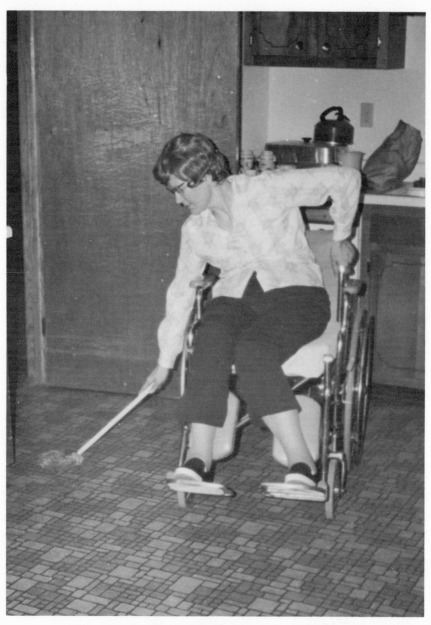

Mopping the floor, using the little mop mentioned
in this chapter and the previous chapter.

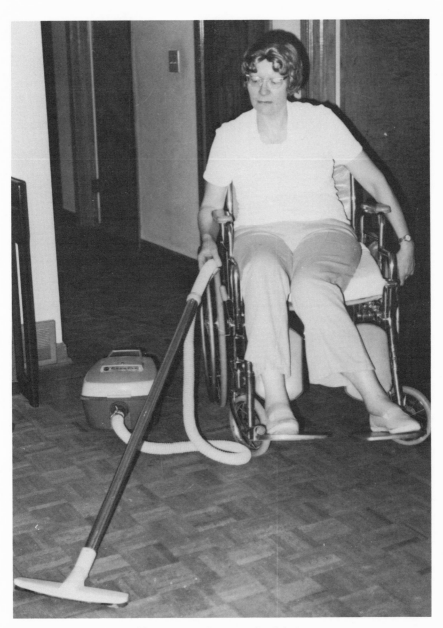

Vacuuming from a wheelchair.

to wash is small, such as a bathroom usually is, you can do the whole thing with the little mop and not bother to get the big one out. Several of these mops would be practical —possibly one for the kitchen, one for the bathroom or one for floors, and one for other jobs. Two pluses about this item: it fits rather inconspicuously in a corner of a room and small children enjoy using it.

Generally, before you wash a floor, you first sweep up the loose dirt. This double chore would not bother anyone with endless energy. However, if you're not strong or if, like me, you have days when you are already exhausted though you've barely begun the day, you might want to try this shortcut. Sometimes I mop, drawing the pieces of leaves, dried mud, and dirt along toward the doorway and frequently rinsing out in a pail as I move along. When I reach the door, my floor is clean and I just sweep (with the mop) the small pile of dirt onto a dustpan and deposit it in a basket.

Waxing the kitchen floor is not something I do often— by the time I get the floor washed, I have very little time, energy or desire to wax it. One way that might make it a little easier is to use a product which cleans and waxes at the same time. To avoid waxing ever, you might consider putting down the type of vinyl flooring that needs no waxing. Even if it costs more, it may be worth the extra expense.

When it comes to wood floors, it is probably most practical to have someone apply paste wax on hands and knees, then rent a floor polisher and buff the floor. Or, from a wheelchair, you can apply liquid polish with a wax applicator.

Vacuuming is one of the most tiring jobs to do from a wheelchair. I think so, anyway, and have talked with others who agree with me. The first thing to consider is how to convey the cleaner. A canister type will probably move more easily if set on a dolly. I drag mine along behind me like a puppy dog on a chain. As I move from one room to another, I keep the hose across my shoulder and between my legs. With one of the removable legs off my chair (crossing my legs at the ankle on the remaining footrest), at times I house the vacuum underneath, letting my chair frame push it along. This is especially good when in small rooms where you can get all wound up in the cord and hose and scarcely find enough space to turn around.

I actually have two vacuums and the second is what they call a lightweight upright. Lightweight it isn't and I get more tired using it than the other. It has no attachments for dusting books or hard-to-reach corners so for these things I use the other one.

Cleaning under beds and low furniture means bending far down and some people may find this rather hazardous. I hang onto my chair with one hand as I lean over. Although I don't think of it as dangerous for myself, it does tire me more than doing an open floor. Usually I leave these spots to be done by a dustmop, which is much easier to manage, and then only occasionally do them with a vacuum.

There is something you might be interested in if you are living in a permanent home, and by that I mean if you own your own house and do not expect to be moving in the near future—a built-in vacuum system. With this, there is no cleaner to move about, just a long hose. They are generally quiet to operate and need only to be emptied after many, many months—no bags involved. Of course, in comparison to going to the store and buying a vacuum cleaner, this is an expensive proposition; yet it might not be in the long run. It certainly is more convenient and adds to the resale value of your home. If you would like to learn more about the built-in system, look in the yellow pages of your telephone book for places to contact in your town. You can also find them described in a Sears catalogue.

There are two substitutes for a vacuum. One is called a hand or carpet sweeper. These are fine for removing surface dirt quickly but they are wide and will not go into narrow places. All of them will sweep a carpet but only the ones that specify they will also clean bare floors can be relied on to do this. This type has a switch which adjusts the brush level for floor or carpet use.

A dustmop is another device that can be used instead of a vacuum, although, like the broom, it doesn't do as thorough a job. They are light to handle and can easily get into spots that, if done with a vacuum, require much twisting and bending. I have two heads for mine and can put a clean one on when the other gets too dirty. Then I take my time getting around to washing the soiled one.

To ease the floor-cleaning job, the dirt can be pulled from under furniture into the center of the room and then "eaten up" by a vacuum. Another way is to make dustmopping the general routine while a more thorough job is done with a vacuum at less frequent intervals by you or someone else.

8

LAUNDRY

If your laundry area is in the basement at the bottom of fourteen steps or outside in a storeroom which you couldn't possibly get into with a wheelchair, you obviously cannot do the washing. On the other hand, many modern homes have the laundry area in or near the kitchen. The first part of this chapter is for those who are able to wash their laundry. After that I talk about ironing which you might be able to do whether or not you have a hand in the washing.

You can save much time and trouble ironing by carefully selecting permanent press clothes for yourself and the family. The combination of these clothes and modern washers and dryers with a permanent press cycle on them can virtually eliminate that hated chore of ironing. A good way to accumulate permanent press clothes is to replace every ironable piece that is destined for the give-away bag or rag pile with those made of permanent press. Also, tell those who buy gifts of clothes for you or for members of your family that you want only permanent press, to make it easier for you. People are usually cooperative that way.

The first job in washing, of course, is bringing the clothes from the hamper—which is usually kept in the bathroom—to the washer. Tall hampers make it quite hard to reach in and get clothes. A shorter one, about twenty inches high, is the kind the wheelchair user needs.

There are a number of ways to carry clothes. You can pile a load on a lapboard. Another sensible approach is to use a laundry cart on casters which can be shoved along in front of you as you wheel. Some of these have a shelf underneath which can be used for folded items after they are dried. There is also a sorter cart with several compartments. These carts fold flat when not in use and can be bought wherever laundry equipment is sold.

Here are other suggestions for carting laundry. You can have a laundry bag set in the hamper. Clothes go right into the bag and at wash time you just lift it out and carry it on your lap. Clothes may be piled into a dishpan which you keep on the floor of the linen closet just for that purpose. These pans cannot be filled too high unless you want to leave a trail of socks and panties behind you. Stuffing soiled laundry in an old pillow case is the method that suits me best. To eliminate the job of sorting colored and white clothes, I have a piece of stiff cardboard down the middle of the hamper to separate them.

A hamper doesn't *have* to be in the bathroom, of course. It may work better for you to have a small hamper in several different places around the house. If you use something lightweight for a hamper, such as a plastic laundry basket, and set it up on something fairly level with your chair, you can pick the container up and carry it to the washer. There might be a spot close to the washer where you can keep the hamper and thus avoid carting your clothes from one place to another. Various family members can have a temporary container for soiled clothes in their bedrooms and then bring their things to such hampers in the morning. This is the sort of thing you have to decide for yourself. Only you know your needs, capabilities, and house space.

Many people keep soiled diapers in a dry pail, sometimes with a deodorant cake inside. I always kept them in water with some type of disinfectant in it. Those of you who also do this will find a pail filled with soggy diapers and water mighty heavy. It certainly is not something which can be balanced on a lap during the trip from bathroom to washer. This is a good thing to leave for another person to lift and carry for you. You can keep the pail on a dolly and just push it in front of your chair or have the pail near the washer, but it will still need to be lifted and dumped into the washer. There is one thing you can do by yourself, though. Several times when I was in need of diapers and my husband wasn't home to lift the pail for me, I managed to put half the diapers into an empty pail and then lift both pails onto my lapboard. The best thing to do, I suppose, is to use the other method of keeping diapers.

Now that you are at the washer, where are you going to keep supplies? Naturally, detergent, bleach, pre-soak, fabric softener, and whatever else you use has to be within reach. You may have a cabinet nearby in which to keep everything. I have a small shelf over my dryer for such things. It has to be over the dryer because such a shelf must be low in order for me to reach it. It could not have been placed over my top-loading washer—not if I wanted to be able to open the lid of the machine. My most frequently used supplies are on a small turntable so they are always at my fingertips.

Once your clothes are washed, your next task is to get them dried. There are lots of people who think that hanging clothes outdoors is the only right way to do it. Whether or not you can hang your clothes outside depends on if you are able to get in and out of the house by yourself. If you have to go down a ramp to get to the clothesline, it seems to me that pushing a cartful of clothes in front of you could be disastrous. Perhaps you could have a clothesline or drying rack in a more convenient spot, such as a carport. Just the thing for such a purpose is a square steel outdoor clothes dryer which adjusts in height, as advertised in a Sears catalogue.

As far as I am concerned, there never has been a better way to dry clothes than by using a dryer. They certainly make life easier for the wheelchair housekeeper. If you haven't bought any laundry appliances yet, and want to avoid switching clothes from washer to dryer, you can start with a washer-dryer combination.

A word about dryers. We used to have an old type with a rather narrow door and there was room enough to pull up close to the door, pull it part-way down and reach into the dryer. Then we got a new one which has a door the entire width of the machine. It has the type of door which will slam shut if not pulled down all the way. If I open the

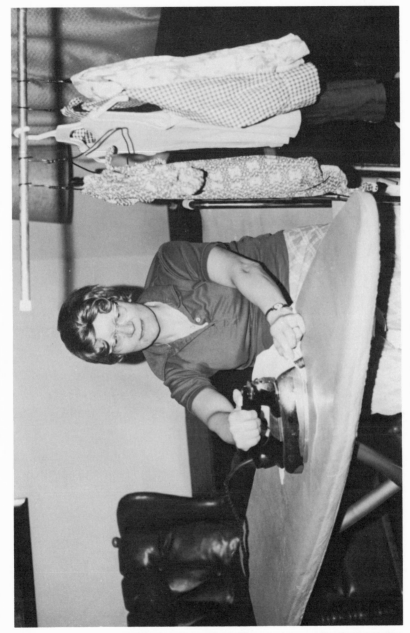

Ironing, with the ironing rack next to the board.

door all the way, though, much of my laundry is too far from me, so I use one of the aids I mentioned in an earlier chapter.

Permanent press should be taken out of the dryer at the end of a cycle and hung immediately. You can eliminate even more ironing by taking all clothes out of the dryer as soon as it stops. Many nonpermanent press materials will look presentable if handled like their more modern closet-mates. However, if a batch of clothes gets wrinkled because it wasn't taken out in time, it can be put through a rinse cycle in the washer and returned to the dryer.

I am not the only one in a wheelchair whose hands are partially or completely numb. So how do you test clothes for dryness when you cannot rely on your hands? I do this by rubbing them against my cheek. I have to laugh when my youngest does this. Apparently she thinks this is the proper way since Mama does it!

Whether you like the job or not, folding clothes takes time. With six in my family, it seems I am forever plowing through mounds of sheets, towels, and socks. I toss the clothes to be ironed from the dryer into a bag, and leave the rest dumped on my bed or the kitchen table. Then I go around the house doing other things and make up my mind to fold a certain number of pieces every time I go into the bedroom, even if it is only to get a tissue to blow my nose or to put on some lipstick. I make up a similar rule when the clothes are on the table. Eventually, the mountain of laundry disappears.

Ironing from a wheelchair is not the most desirable job in the world. However, everyone has some clothes that need ironing. Even if you use permanent press, there will be times when you didn't get the clothes out of the dryer right after the cycle finished and they got wrinkled. Or perhaps you don't have the advantage of a dryer at all. Even new clothes need a little ironing to get out the lines caused from being folded in packages.

In order to iron, of course, you start with an ironing board, nowadays called an ironing table. The height of modern boards is adjustable to several levels so it is not difficult to set them at a level that is comfortable when used from a seated position. If you have an area where you can leave your board permanently set up, that is ideal. If you must keep your board in a closet and get it out for each use, it will be a good idea to have casters put on the bottom of the legs to insure easy rolling. Getting the board out might be a job to reserve for someone other than you.

Okay, the board is set up. Now you have to assemble all your supplies—your container of clothes to be done, spray starch, hangers, and whatever else you ordinarily use to make the job as painless as possible. For hanging clothes after ironing, you will probably need a laundry rack, sometimes called a caddy or valet, and available wherever ironing equipment is sold. The height is adjustable and some come with a flatwork shelf and ironing supplies basket. These racks are very lightweight and fold flat for storage.

Before you iron, let me issue a warning: *be careful!* I once came close to burning myself badly with a steam iron. I had finished ironing a shirt, set the iron on the board, and with the shirt in one hand, wheeled my chair just a little with the other hand to get closer to the rack and hang the shirt. Then I did what I had always been afraid I would do —caught the iron cord on my wheel and yanked the plug out of the wall. Luckily, the iron fell on the floor rather than my lap. If you are going to move away from the board, always check first to see that the cord is not caught on your chair. A cord minder to keep the cord from tangling can prevent a disaster. Check in an ironing supplies department of a store for this.

One thing I have always found troublesome at the height we have to work is that shirtsleeves sweep the floor. To avoid this, you can lay some newspapers or an old sheet on the floor. Also, a chair or other piece of furniture can be placed in front of the board on which clothes hang down.

Another thing, in your standing-up days you probably pulled the article being ironed toward you. Learn to reverse this method. If you pull the clothes toward you, they will end up in your lap getting all crumpled and defeating your purpose.

Instead of going through the trouble of setting up an ironing table, you might want to try using a card table covered with something quite heavy such as several thicknesses of a folded mattress pad. This will give you a large working area and you will have no trouble getting your legs underneath it but you will not have a narrow open end such as you find on an ironing table.

When there's only a small amount of touch-up ironing to be done, here are two suggestions. First, use a portable or travel ironing board. This can be used on something like the kitchen table. Or use a lapboard with a heavy mattress pad, folded several times, on top of it. The board will have to be well padded or the heat of the iron will take off the finish of the board. (You will never guess how I found that out!) There's no room on the board for the iron so you must arrange to set it on something next to you as you work.

Either of these methods is good for putting iron-on patches on clothes.

One other word about ironing. If you have daughters, I heartily recommend that you teach them to iron as early in their life as you think reasonable. Naturally, this has to be well supervised at first, but once they learn to do it they can relieve you of much of the work.

9
CHILD
CARE

There is one thing you would do well to remember about taking care of children from a wheelchair: live one day at a time and handle problems *as they arise.* There is no sense, for instance, in losing sleep worrying about how you will handle your six-months-old child when he begins to walk. He may be a late walker and the situation won't even have to be faced for many months. Then, too, a child doesn't all of a sudden leap up from bed and begin walking. First he learns to sit up by himself. Then he may or may not go through the crawling stage. Certainly before he's exploring the house on foot he will pull up to a stand and start walking around the bed or playpen. In other words, you will have plenty of warning. When the time does seem to be approaching, then make your preparations and start planning strategy.

Since I have four children, I don't think I can be accused

of sitting at a desk and writing a lot of advice off the top of my head. As in all areas of this book, I try to offer methods with which I am personally familiar or those I know others have used. However, everything about infant care is, of necessity, not derived from personal experience since I was not physically able to care for my youngest child until she was well past her first birthday.

A tiny baby needs to be fed, changed, bathed, and dressed and that is really about all. Let's say that the little one has been fast asleep in his crib and awakens with hunger pangs. You will first want to change him, but to park next to his bed and change and dress him sideways isn't comfortable for most people. What you really need is an all-purpose table, preferably on casters to be moved easily, one that will be level with the crib when the rail is down, with space under it for your legs so you can work in a forward position. This can have drawers on the side for diapers, clothes and other supplies, or you can have a low chest next to the table for this purpose. Using such a table, the child can be transferred fairly easily from the crib into a convenient position for you. If you cannot lift the child over, you can put a sliding board between bed and table, making sure, of course, that any board you use is smooth and without splinters. This table will probably have to be especially built. In order for it to be built correctly, explain to the person making it exactly what you need.

One more word about that table, should you decide to have one made. If you think it is too much trouble and expense to go into for the short time it would be needed, you might like to know that it comes in very handy long

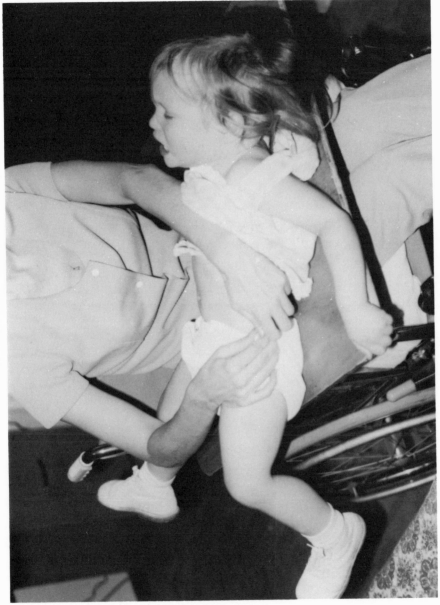

Changing a baby on a lapboard.

after the baby is through with it. It can be used for typing, cutting out patterns, art work, and just about anything you might use a table for. If you have it made with drawers, it makes a perfect desk afterward.

Rather than a special table for baby care, a table meant for a portable sewing machine might be ideal. Of course, the only way to find out is to try it.

What I found useful for diapering an older baby would be even more advantageous for a young one—that old standby, the lapboard. What I liked about using it was that you have the baby right in front of you where you can get a good grip on him to prevent his rolling off.

As I said before, a board can be used to bridge the gap between the crib and any dressing surface you use. This is only necessary when the baby is quite young. Children of handicapped mothers seem to have a built-in mechanism for catching on to ways that make life easier for everybody. At a young age, they learn to make the transfer by themselves.

After solving the problem of getting the baby in a position to be changed, the actual diapering has to be faced. For those who do not have full use of their hands, this isn't so simple, but there are a number of ways to overcome the obstacle. For instance, when I first began taking care of my youngest, pins were unmanageable for me. So I bought some terry-cloth-lined plastic pants and put a diaper between her legs before pulling on the pants. It worked for me.

Two more possible solutions for someone who cannot handle a safety pin are snap-on diapers and diaper pants. The first is a diaper which snaps together without pins. They are not available just anywhere so you will have to inquire about local sources or obtain them through the large mail-order catalogues, such as Sears. The second—diaper pants—are heavy since they are made especially for night wear, but they are suitable for a large or older baby of over twenty pounds.

Diapering can be eased by Velcro, a nylon tape fastener which requires no pins. It can be sewn on a diaper in a horizontal position, one half on the back of a diaper, the other in the place which would ordinarily be pinned over it, allowing for the growth of the baby. More details about Velcro can be found in the discussion of clothing in the chapter on personal grooming.

The same advantages will be found in the disposable diapers made with tape that remain together without pins.

When the little guy is comfortably dry, it is time for him to eat. The mother who nurses her baby eliminates some problems here. Nowadays, however, the majority of babies are bottle-fed. If the baby is only going to get a bottle at this time, he can be left in bed while you heat up the bottle and then take it into the bedroom and feed him. When there are going to be some solids, too, you will probably want to bring him into the kitchen to eat his meal. Obviously, you cannot hold a child and wheel your chair at the same time. You can carry him in an infant seat, attaching the strap to your chair and then feeding him right in the seat on your lap. Another idea that might appeal to you is to strap an automobile seat belt to the frame of your chair. When not in use, your belt will lay beside you on the seat. Then when you want to carry your child, the belt fastens around both of you. You can also use a belt of some other kind, as long as it is long and strong enough.

Now we are ready to discuss bathing. If your special-made table has a dressing table portion that lifts up with a tub underneath it for bathing, that will be especially helpful. You might consider including this feature when you have the table built. You can push the table to the kitchen or bathroom to fill the tub with a spray or shampoo hose. Another person can empty the water later.

The woman who cared for my baby before I was able to gave her a bath in the kitchen sink. If you have a sink which you can get your legs under, this might be convenient for you. There generally is a counter on one or both sides of the sink where the baby can be set down to towel off and dress, and the sink can be scoured out after each use. When I no longer needed full-time help and my baby was older, I had one of the older children get in the tub with her to see that she was well scrubbed and wouldn't slip. (I like to let the kids have bubble bath in their water to help get them clean without much effort and to avoid a bathtub ring.) If there are no older children to rely on, maybe this can be left for Daddy to do. There are some mothers who want to bathe by themselves a child old enough to sit up in a tub alone. As I've mentioned before, a footstool, or something else low, could make it less difficult for her to get from chair to floor and back.

When it comes to a playpen, it is best to have one which raises up to the height of a wheelchair, such as a portable crib, or the type with a drop side which can be made level with your chair. The object, of course, is to make the child reachable. Again, a sliding board can be used, this time between chair and playpen and back.

Parents of a crawling or walking baby usually go around the house childproofing—temporarily putting breakables out of the reach of little hands, surveying all areas for possibility of danger, putting such items as cleaning supplies somewhere other than under the sink, or padlocking the cabinet, and covering electrical outlets with those gadgets you can get at a hardware store to prevent children from poking things into them. A wheelchair mother ought to be extra careful about these things. She cannot run to rescue a child from calamity as the lady next door can. Any sections of the house which are forbidden to the child and are also impossible for the mother to get into should have a portable safety gate in front of them, at least during the day when others are not around to help. There are several different types of these gates and they are found where baby equipment is sold. Also, doors of rooms the child should not enter can be kept locked.

Do your fingers misbehave when they meet with short shoestrings, such as are found on children's shoes? If so, there are several things you can do. One is to see that the child is up in the morning before others leave the house for work or school, so they can tie the shoes for you. Or have an understanding with a neighbor who will come over at a specified time daily to do this job. Have them double knot the strings to keep them from opening. To avoid the problem at naptime, let the child sleep with his shoes on. Another thing you can do, if you have your pediatrician's approval, is get the child into buckled or slip-on shoe styles as soon as possible.

Besides diaper pins and shoestrings, many people find that the tiny buttons on a little girl's dress or boy's shirt are impossible or at least frustrating to manage. This hurdle can also be jumped. Infants can wear slip-on and zip-up

119

clothes or, as described in the chapter on personal grooming, Velcro can be sewn into their clothes. Somewhat older preschoolers can take care of the button front pieces themselves with a little assistance to line up the buttons with the proper buttonholes. Playwear is often something as simple as pullon pants and pullover shirts, which are no trouble for children. Those button-back dresses, which neither you nor a little girl can handle, can be set aside until someone else is there to help.

The wheelchair mother who has a fenced yard has some peace of mind when it comes to letting a toddler go outside alone. If you must let him go out in an unfenced yard, you can keep an eye on him better if you are able to get in and out of the house yourself. Still, that is no advantage if he won't come to you. I believe that even very young children should be taught the importance of coming when you call. If you stress, "I *can't* go and look for you. You *must* come when I call," they soon get the message.

Even if you have a very obedient child, it is a good idea to check on him often. If you don't see or hear him for a while, call. Also, your neighbors know that you cannot chase up and down the street for kids who have wandered off. You might ask some of the ones nearby to let you know if they see your children in forbidden territory.

Older children, when they are home, can be responsible for looking after preschoolers but I don't think it is fair to expect them to keep it up for hours at a time.

If you have no older children, live on a heavily traveled street and don't trust your child on his own, he can still get some fresh air while you keep your nerves intact. Let him be a predominantly indoors child until he reaches a more dependable age. I don't mean that you should never let him go out—just don't allow him out when you are the only person available to look after him. His father can take him outdoors for as long as possible in the evening, perhaps while he trims the bushes or picks up clutter on the lawn. Or a grandmother, aunt or friend can take the child out now and then or at certain times of the week. There might be a teenager in the neighborhood who is glad to earn a little money by taking your child outside for a specified length of time each nice day. There are, of course, going to be cold and rainy days when all children stay in. Time is in your favor because, more quickly than you realize, that small child won't be so small anymore. Limited outdoor life, of itself, does not make a sickly child. My youngest girl spent a great amount of time inside until I could be more sure of her actions, and she has always been very healthy.

It is wise parents who teach their young children independence at an early age. While still babies, children of a wheelchair mother can hang on to their mother while she uses her hands to wheel. At a time when other youngsters depend on their mothers to dress them, these children take care of themselves quite well *if you let them*. A preschooler can get his clothes up and down from closets providing the bar is low enough. You can get an extension bar that fits onto the regular closet rod, some of which are adjustable in height. Look for them where closet accessories are sold. The young child can get clothes out of drawers that are low enough to reach and can dress and undress himself. He may not be able to tie his shoes but a little girl can buckle hers.

I personally believe that the more independent your children are, the better for all concerned. Of course, by that I don't mean leaving them completely without supervision. Here is an example of what I mean. There are times when I am not able to get into the kitchen before my children leave for school. That means that I don't get to see what kind of atrocious color combinations they may be wearing. But I don't worry about them because, on a school morning, my kids can get along fine on their own. Breakfast is juice and cereal and sometimes toast, which they can prepare themselves, even if they do usually make a mess. They get dressed, and if it is anyone's day to change his sheets, that too is done. They sometimes make their lunches the night before, put the perishables in the refrigerator and assemble everything in the morning, or they do it all in the morning. So I know they can get along without me.

Sometimes you must rely on children more than you originally planned. I began letting my oldest daughter learn a few things about cooking simply because she showed interest. As I write this, however, there have been times when it was necessary for me to issue instructions for making supper while I laid on the bed—and I was grateful she was able to carry them out.

10

PERSONAL GROOMING

Most people can get ready for the day at home or away without much effort. For the handicapped, dressing can be a major project. Sometimes, though, people experience difficulty because they don't know of a method which would ease the process. Hopefully, this section will contain at least a few helpful ideas for wheelchair users.

I like to wear clothes that are easy to get in and out of. Like most women I know, I often wear slacks around the house. The kinds with the elastic waistband (no zipper) are easy to pull on and are most practical for me since I seem to make a hobby of collecting broken zippers. With these pants, ordinary blouses can be worn. The simplest top to wear is the pullover shirt or sweater—no buttons. This would also be true for men. However, the person who has limited motion in the arms and cannot get his or her hands overhead to pull on a shirt or sweater will not consider it so ideal. Buttons might be better for such people. If neither a pullover top or a buttoned one will do, how about snap or zipper closings which can be sewn into clothes?

Without being aware of it, you may be familiar with another answer for those who cannot manage buttons. If you have had your blood pressure taken and the instrument was strapped to your arm, then later peeled off, that was Velcro. This same fastener can be sewn into the closing of a blouse, shirt, dress or skirt instead of buttons or zippers. This item now also comes in an iron-on version. Velcro is a double strip of nylon tape, usually about three-quarters inches wide, each side of which has a different texture. The two are pressed together to close, pulled apart to open. It comes in neutral colors such as white, black, or beige and is sold by the yard at fabric shops.

Some people may have no trouble at all getting completely dressed in a wheelchair. As for me, anything that I have to put on over my head or put my arms through, I do in the chair because if I do it on the bed, I'm easily overbalanced and topple over. When I have the top part of me dressed, I get on the bed to put on my pants, socks, and shoes with laces.

Poor balance can really make getting dressed difficult. I am definitely speaking from experience. Putting on pants, hose, or braces can be at least a little easier if it is done while you're sitting up against the headboard of the bed, or with something at your back such as one of those wedge-shaped cushions that are designed for watching TV or reading in bed. Some of them have arms on either side with a handy pocket on each. They are called a bedrest and are found where spreads or cushions are sold.

Those who are able to sit Indian fashion will find that this is a way to maintain balance when dressing on the bed. For slacks and hose, one leg can be tended to, then the legs crossed in the opposite position and the second one given attention. You pull the pants or hose up to the knee and when both legs are ready, lie down and get them up the rest of the way.

Another method is to sit in your wheelchair to do the job, your feet on the bed. Crossing the legs while sitting in the chair will bring them closer to you.

Underwear is hard for some women to put on. Those who cannot fasten a bra behind them may find that doing it in front is the answer. I put mine on backwards, hook it in front of me and then twist it around the proper way and get my arms under the straps. For those who must work with one hand, Velcro can be sewn where the bra fastens.

Around the house in the morning or evening, many women like to wear a robe or duster. I find it convenient to wear mine backwards and have someone button me up in the back. Worn that way, they do not have to be buttoned all the way or tucked down completely under you either. Another advantage—you stay decently covered in front. Robes and dusters which zip all the way up the front can be bought as well as some outfits for home use that have snap fronts.

For a woman, getting dressed to go somewhere can be a little more complicated than dressing for home. Dressier clothes seem automatically to mean zippers or buttons in the back. That is not hard to overcome, though. A person who is home with you while you get ready can take care of this one phase of your dressing, or if a woman is picking you up, you can save the job for her. If there is no one to rely on but yourself, you just have to be selective when buying clothes. Always buy garments that open in front. Large buttons are easier to handle than small ones. You may find it a help to button a dress partway while it is in front of you on your lap or the table, leaving just enough open at the top to get it over your head. Zippered-front dresses can save a lot of frustration. They're not abundant in "going places" clothes but they are around if you watch newspapers and catalogues. If this is the kind you like, it might be a good idea, when you do come across them, to buy several different styles and colors. If a dress or blouse isn't too tight, it can often be put over the head and the back opening zipped or buttoned in front of you, then turned around and your arms put in.

For a catalogue of clothes especially made for the handicapped woman, write to Fashion-Able, Inc.

When I am getting dressed to go somewhere, I put on my slip, dress, or skirt and blouse while in the chair. I get all buttoned and zipped but do not bother to pull everything down straight. Then I get on the bed and put on my stockings. For some, panty hose is the perfect kind to wear. I prefer the type which are elasticized up to the top of the thigh, needing no garters. They are available most places where hose is sold. After I get these on, I lie down and roll from side to side while pulling my clothes down to a proper position.

Unless a person can stand up, full length coats are a nuisance to get tucked down. The only short ones you can usually find, however, are the casual type, which you might not care to wear for every occasion. If you do get a long coat, try to get one as unbulky as possible.

Large purses are clumsy to carry for a woman who does a lot of wheeling. Since both her hands are occupied, the purse has to set on her lap and may find its way to the floor a time or two. Of course, this doesn't apply to a woman small enough to have the space to prop a purse next to her on the chair. You may, like me, have room next to you for a fairly flat purse rather than those wide, hefty kind, so keep that in mind when you are ready to buy a new purse.

A word about shoes. Slip-on styles can be exasperating to wear as they are inclined to fall off when you transfer. Buckled or tied shoes are more likely to stay put. When I am going somewhere and want to wear a slip-on style, I just carry the shoes along until I get out of the car at my destination and then put them on.

Several different types of shoelaces that do not need to be tied can be found in a Cleo Living Aids catalogue.

I used to consider slippers or shoes useless to wear around the house and would often go about barefoot. I have changed my mind. Since my feet have no feeling, I am apt to bang my toes without paying any attention to it. Once I collided with the refrigerator and ended up with a huge, purple big toe and couldn't put on a shoe for five days. There was another occurrence and I get slightly ill thinking about it (I'd make the world's worst nurse). I pulled off a whole toenail without being aware of it until I got ready for bed and discovered a bloody toe. If you lack feeling in your feet, I recommend that you allow your toes to be bare only when you are fairly certain they will not be damaged, such as when in the tub, bed, or wide-open spaces.

Confinement to a wheelchair and poor bladder control, or lack of it, often go hand in hand so incontinent pants are the next topic. They can be bought at various surgical and rehabilitation supply houses in your vicinity or through mail-order catalogues offering this type of merchandise. Several different styles are described and pictured in a Cleo Living Aids catalogue and even a Sears catalogue has some under sickroom supplies. That's the most I can say since this is a personal problem for which a really satisfactory solution has not yet been found.

Nowadays, combing, setting and styling hair need not be difficult because of limited use of the hands. Little care is needed if hair is worn very short. If not that, consider a wig, which is fashionable and reasonably priced.

Uncapping a lipstick is a major project for some women. However, it takes far less strength to pull off the cap if it isn't pushed on tightly when closed. When there is only one hand to work with, thus making the turning up of the lipstick the problem, you can leave the cap off and the lipstick permanently turned up and kept in a plastic sandwich bag.

Getting close to a regular dresser or bathroom mirror is not possible from a wheelchair so a hand mirror is a real necessity for combing hair or putting on lipstick. One with a plastic handle, which is made to bend, can be set on a table by itself and doesn't need to be held. Then if your hand is unsteady with a tube of lipstick in it, you can rest your elbow on the table. This mirror is also helpful for a man using an electric shaver. Then, there are more expensive stand-up mirrors that light up. These are usually called make-up mirrors.

11

MISCELLANEOUS

There are some aspects of wheelchair life that do not fit into any of the previous chapters of this book. Therefore, it seemed sensible to me to reserve them for the final chapter.

You probably already know that you can save some of your "wheeling energy" if you pull along doorways or pieces of furniture with one hand as you move about. It also can speed your trips around the house. For instance, you can pull on anything that won't fall over or open up when you do it, such as the doorknob of a closed door, the handle of a heavy chest, a sink, the side of the refrigerator, an end of a dresser or edge of a table.

Even if the household arrangements in your present home work out well for you, a change of furniture or house may present problems you did not previously have. For example, I had a floor lamp that, with some stretching, I could turn on and off by myself. Then we got rid of it and bought end tables and table lamps, which made a rearrangement of furniture necessary. As a result, one lamp was out of my reach. Now we have made both lamps work off the wall switch so I can turn them off together. If I need just a little light in the room, I can turn off the reachable lamp.

I have already issued a warning for people who have no sensation in their feet. Here's another. If someone runs bath water for you, tell him to test it before you get in or if you fill the tub yourself, be sure to do this. People lacking sensation generally cannot even tell if it's water, let alone if it is hot or cold.

Lack of feeling can create a problem in another way. One time I spilled coffee, just poured out of the pot, on my knee. Although my leg jerked in a violent spasm, I felt nothing and ignored it. Since I was wearing pants, I couldn't see what had happened. It was not until I undressed for bed that I discovered the spilled coffee had resulted in blisters which broke open and bled. I still have a scar on my knee today. What I am trying to say is—do check on a possible injury even if you don't feel it. You could be more badly hurt than you realize.

I always thought of myself as fairly independent until one day when my husband took the kids on an overnight camping trip. They left on the morning of one day and returned on the evening of the next. While we were making preparations for this trip, I was not at all concerned about staying home alone. All that would be necessary, I thought, was to have a list of neighbors' phone numbers handy in case they were needed, which I already had anyway. Then my husband remembered that I couldn't get the food dish to feed our dog, who is housed in our fenced-in backyard. So he arranged that a neighbor's children would get the food pan for me and then return the full one outside, giving our pooch some water at the same time. Feeding the dog seemed to be the only difficulty. It wasn't. I discovered that our rural-type mailbox was very hard for me to handle, and getting the morning paper from the front lawn wasn't too easy either. Ordinarily, my husband or children tend to these chores. My neighbor's children enjoyed doing the little jobs of helping care for the dog and bringing me my mail and paper. On the other hand, I realized that for some things I am very much dependent upon others and I must be grateful for the assistance I receive whenever necessary.

Many people enjoy gardening. There are some things which can be done from a seated position, such as trimming bushes. You can also try weeding with a tongs from a chair. But for actual digging and planting, the only practical method is to get out of the wheelchair and sit on the ground. People who are able to stand or have the strength to pull themselves back into the chair from the ground might try this. For those who need assistance to get in and out of the wheelchair, the outdoor work should be done when someone is there to help. If you are going to do this alone, remember to assemble your equipment beforehand. It can be quite irritating to get yourself settled on the ground, ready to begin work, and then discover you have forgotten your trowel.

Those who find regular outdoor gardening too much to handle but love that type of work might consider indoor

133

gardening activities. All types of window shelves, flower carts, and wagons are available from mail order firms, trading stamp companies, and local department stores.

Regardless of the method used, tub bathing is too difficult for some. You know, in the hospital you take a so-called bath every day from a little pan of water. At home, you can take what I call installment plan baths. I call them that because you wash the upper half of you at the sink and then you (or someone else) with a lapboard on your chair carries a pan of water to the bed where you wash the bottom half.

Typing may not be a tiring task for everyone, but it is for some, including myself. I have found two methods of dealing with this exhaustion. One is that after typing for a while, I do something else or lie down for a few minutes, returning later to type some more. Since sometimes I cannot sit at the typewriter at all and on other days I feel fairly good, my second method is to type a lot on my better days to make up for the idle ones.

Where you use a typewriter makes a difference in your performance. Whether or not you can get close to one which is set on a standard typing table depends upon your type of chair. With nondetachable legrests, you can sit kitty-corner with one foot on each side of one of the table's legs. With swing-away legrests, you can either move them aside or take them off completely, and put your feet on the floor, thus getting as close to the table as anyone possibly can. Short people may not be able to touch the floor with their feet, though. Even middle-height people may find space between their feet and the floor if they are sitting on a regular wheelchair cushion, which makes you higher in the chair. This can be remedied by removing the cushion while you type or by putting something such as a telephone book under your feet.

You can keep a typewriter on a desk rather than a typing table. Standard desks are not suitable for wheelchairs since the leg space is generally too narrow. (Of course, to get under a desk at all, you need desk arms on your chair). I made a very adequate desk out of two two-drawer filing cabinets with a five-foot-long plywood board laid across the top and plenty of leg space between the cabinets. The board can be any length you wish and stained and varnished or painted, and the distance between the cabinets is up to you. This places a typewriter in a much higher position than when it's on a typing table, though, and puts more strain on the arms. It helps to sit on something to make yourself higher in the chair. I often put another wheelchair cushion on top of the one I always have in the chair.

Holding onto a phone requires more strength than some people have. To carry on conversations with ease, what they need is a shoulder phone rest which enables a person to talk on the phone without hanging onto it every minute. These can be bought through various mail-order catalogues but you can also get one at your local office supplies store.

If your hand is unsteady and you find brushing your teeth a problem, try doing it a different way. Lean your elbow against the bathroom washbowl and, instead of moving your hand back and forth, move your head back and forth.

Let me put in a word for something which can be done

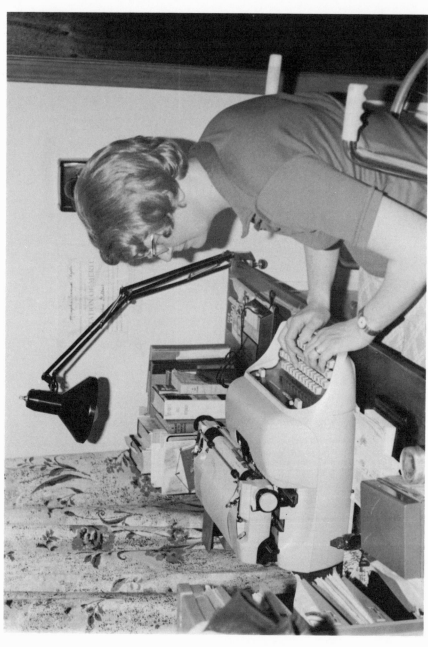

Typing.

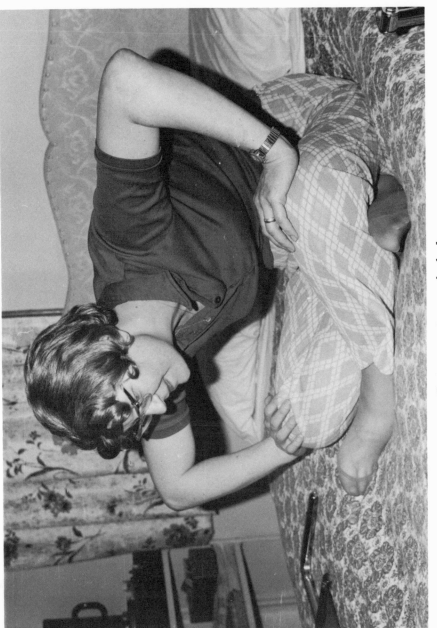

Doing exercises on the bed.

at home and from a wheelchair—writing. An editor doesn't care whether you can walk or not or how much schooling you have had either. He is only interested in how well you write. I did a smattering of writing in my "walking days" but far more since I've been forced to sit all the time. If you have talent in that direction, nothing beats it for getting your mind off yourself.

People in wheelchairs ought to exercise daily to compensate for the lack of movement and activity necessitated by their confinement to a chair. Naturally, what you can or should do is entirely dependent upon your capabilities and your doctor's instructions. To me, the most practical place to exercise is on the bed. Please do not do anything at the edge of a bed which might possibly cause you to fall on the floor. Anything that would mean a lot of movement can be done more safely on an exercise mat on the floor. Sit-ups are a recommended exercise for many people but maybe they are impossible for you to do on your own. In a physical therapy department, they often give you a dumbbell to hold in each hand to help bring you forward. At home, I use two plastic bottles filled with wet sand.

Some people can do a limited amount of walking between the parallel bars in a therapy department but are deprived of this when they are at home. Doctors will tell you that even a short period of walking each day is better for you than constantly sitting. You can have those bars at home for considerably less than they are sold commercially. Mine are on our carport and are fourteen feet long but, of course, they can be any length you want. The following explanation plus a look at Figure 4 will give you a clearer picture of how they are made.

138

Say you only want eight-foot-long bars. What you need, then, is (1) two eight-foot lengths of one-inch pipe, threaded at both ends; (2) four elbows to go over the ends of the above pipes; (3) four supporting pieces of one-inch pipe, threaded on both ends (see below for length); and (4) four flanges to go at the bottom of each supporting pipe.

The supporting pipes can be any length from the ground that is most convenient for you. To find out, measure the height of anything which is comfortable for you to pull onto and seems to be at the right level for you. To give you some idea: my supporting pipes were made three feet long and I am five-feet seven-inches tall. How far apart the bars should be set is determined by what your size requires and, of course, the space you have to work with. Mine are twenty inches apart.

Now if you want longer bars, such as the fourteen-feet-long ones mine are, you will need (1) four seven-foot lengths of one-inch pipe, threaded at both ends; (2) four elbows to go over the ends of the above pipes; (3) six supporting pieces of one-inch pipe, threaded at both ends (the length you require); (4) two T-pipes to hold each two lengths of pipe together; and (5) six flanges.

The only thing about the bars I have not discussed is bolting down the flanges. A different method is used if they are being put into wood than if they are bolted to concrete. If you are interested in this project, I suggest you seek the assistance of a hardware store man in your area. Or you might seek the help of someone who knows a lot about building such things.

If you put such bars up on the outside, there may be some wintry days when you will want to use them. Many

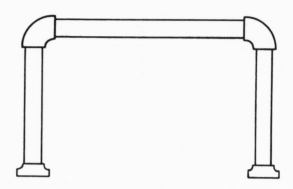

A. Short Bars

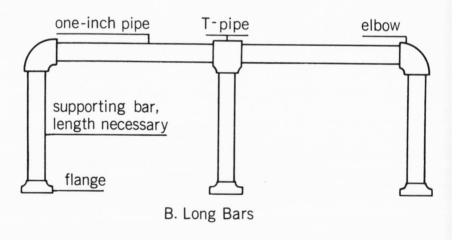

B. Long Bars

Figure 4. Parallel Bars

kinds of gloves will keep your hands warm but if you want a sure grip on the bars, wear leather or driving gloves.

Do you love to read but are unable because of defective vision, difficulty in holding a book or turning pages? The solution to your problem is "Talking Books," which are provided free by the Library of Congress. These are books read by experienced readers—many of whom have a background in radio, television, and movies—recorded on long-playing records, which you play on a record player that is also furnished free. This is the only kind of reading you can do flat on your back with your eyes closed or while dressing, brushing your teeth, mending or dusting. They do not have everything on record but there is quite a bit of variety. Some of the subjects covered include psychology, religion (including the Bible), astronomy, natural history, medical science, biography, poetry, drama, history and fiction—from the classics to *Perry Mason* mysteries. Seven hundred books are issued each year. In addition to books, a number of magazines are on record. If interested in "Talking Books," write to the Division for the Blind and Physically Handicapped, Library of Congress, Washington, D. C. 20542.

The quarterly magazine for the handicapped, *Accent on Living,* was discussed in the introduction to this book. In addition to the advertisements and notices about useful equipment, which I already mentioned, there are articles about, for, and often by handicapped people. I read over my copies again and again. A subscription to this magazine is well worth the price. As usual, see the rear of this book for the address.

Keeping active is tremendous therapy for both physical and emotional well-being. Being active, though, doesn't mean scurrying about the house from one task to another or rushing here and there around town all day. It means, instead, that you forget about the "can'ts" and concentrate on the "cans." For example, playing a game together with your family does not have to involve holding cards with uncooperative hands. There are a lot of dice games. Also, getting away from home for a few hours does not have to involve a lot of transferring in public places, or cost money either. Three occasions that immediately come to my mind are church socials, the opening of a new shopping mall, and a Fourth of July fireworks display.

By now, one thing should be very obvious—there's a great deal that you can do on wheels.

APPENDIX

USEFUL ADDRESSES FOR THE HANDICAPPED

Accent on Living
P. O. Box 726
Bloomington, Ill. 61701

Cleo Living Aids
3957 Mayfield Road
Cleveland, Ohio 44121

Walter Drake
4051 Drake Bldg.
Colorado Springs, Colo.
  80901

Everest and Jennings, Inc.
1803 Pontius Ave.
Los Angeles, Calif. 90025

Fashion-Able, Inc.
Rocky Hill, N. J. 08553

Helen Gallagher-Foster
  House
6523 No. Galena Road
Peoria, Ill. 61601

Gresham Driving Aids
P. O. Box 405A
30800 Wixom Road
Wixom, Mich. 48096

Ted Hoyer and Co. Inc.
2222 Minnesota St.
Oshkosh, Wisc. 54901

Institutional Industries
5500 Muddy Creek Road
Cincinnati, Ohio 45238

Miles Kimball
Oshkosh, Wisc. 54901

National Easter Seals Society
2023 West Ogden Ave.
Chicago, Ill. 60612

National Home Study
  Council
1601 18th St. N. W.
Washington, D. C. 20009

National Hookup
Indoor Sports Club
1255 Val Vista
Pomono, Calif. 91766

National Wheelchair Athletic Association
40–24 62nd St.
Woodside, N. Y. 11377

President's Committee on
  Employment for the
  Handicapped
Washington, D. C. 20210

Rehabilitation Equipment,
  Inc.
175 E. 83 St.
New York, N. Y. 10028

Rolls Equipment Co.
Elyria, Ohio 44035

Wells-Engberg Co., Inc.
2505 Rural St.
Rockford, Ill. 61107

Wheelchair Elevators, Inc.
P. O. Box 489A
Broussard, La. 70518

The Wheelchair Traveler
Ball Hill Road
Milford, N. H. 03055